Georgian Recipes and Remedies

Praise for other titles by Michael J. Rochford

Wakefield Then & Now: Extraordinary Tales from the Merrie City

Escaped bears, out-of-control hot air balloons and tales of secret passages – this book has it all. Rochford's enthusiasm for his home city is evident in this book, which combines folklore and lively stories with fascinating historical detail. *Wakefield Then & Now* paints an intriguing picture of a changing cityscape that you'll want to explore too.
Who Do You Think You Are? Magazine, November 2016

A different Pen and Sword series, 'then and now', this one centring on Wakefield, and providing some terrific local colour and interest for people from the area. Brilliant.
Books Monthly, November 2016

Tales From the Big House: Nostell Priory

Now looked after by the National Trust, the house is visited by many thousands each year, and it is fitting that the quality of workmanship of Robert Adam and Thomas Chippendale displayed inside is matched by Rochford's book. Well and clearly written, much of it based on original correspondence, it is an entertaining read.

Illustrations, which appear throughout the book, are totally relevant, and the list of sources is quite comprehensive considering the book's popular appeal, appearing with rather more description than usual about their use in research on the house's history. In all, a highly recommended book.
Family & Community Historical Research Society

It was with great pleasure and much enthusiasm that I settled down to read Michael Rochford's book *Tales From the Big House: Nostell Priory*.

I found it a very fascinating experience reading about the house I know and love so well through the eyes of someone else and I thoroughly enjoyed every page.

A very well-documented and enjoyable read.

The Lord Charles St. Oswald, September 2019

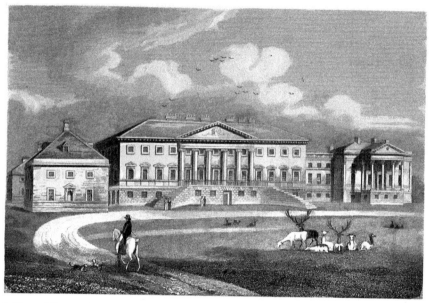

1. Nostell Priory by J.P. Neale, drawn in 1829, from *Views of the Seats, Mansions, Castles etc. of Noblemen and Gentlemen in England, Wales, Scotland and Ireland.*

To Ruth and Christopher Brooks
Thank you for all your love, kindness and support

Georgian Recipes and Remedies

A Country Lady's Household Handbook

Compiled and edited from original source material
by
Michael J. Rochford

with illustrations by
Peter Brears and Caroline Rochford

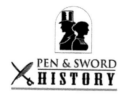

PEN & SWORD
HISTORY

First published in Great Britain in 2020 by
Pen & Sword History
An imprint of
Pen & Sword Books Ltd
Yorkshire – Philadelphia

ISBN 978 1 52672 729 9

A CIP catalogue record for this book is
available from the British Library.

Typeset by Mac Style
Printed and bound in the UK
by CPI Group (UK) Ltd, Croydon, CR0 4YY

Pen & Sword Books Limited incorporates the imprints of Atlas,
Archaeology, Aviation, Discovery, Family History, Fiction, History,
Maritime, Military, Military Classics, Politics, Select, Transport,
True Crime, Air World, Frontline Publishing, Leo Cooper,
Remember When, Seaforth Publishing, The Praetorian Press,
Wharncliffe Local History, Wharncliffe Transport,
Wharncliffe True Crime and White Owl.

For a complete list of Pen & Sword titles please contact

PEN & SWORD BOOKS LIMITED
47 Church Street, Barnsley, South Yorkshire, S70 2AS, England
E-mail: enquiries@pen-and-sword.co.uk
Website: www.pen-and-sword.co.uk

Or

PEN AND SWORD BOOKS
1950 Lawrence Rd, Havertown, PA 19083, USA
E-mail: Uspen-and-sword@casematepublishers.com
Website: www.penandswordbooks.com

Contents

Acknowledgements

I must thank Helen at Wakefield History Centre for granting me permission to transcribe Sabine Winn's receipts, which form part of the fabulous archive of the Winn family of Nostell Priory. My thanks also go to all the staff at Wakefield for their continued assistance and support whenever I visit.

Richard Knowles of Rickaro Books continues to support my projects (not least by stocking my books!) and has sourced useful publications that have assited in my research. He has also offered suggestions for the title of the present work. I'd especially like to thank Richard for his introduction to his great friend, Peter Brears, the food history expert, who has helped enormously with the creation of this book.

I am indebted to Peter for his kind involvement in the project. His book *Gentlewoman's Kitchen: Great Food in Yorkshire 1650–1750* (published by Wakefield Historical Society in 1984) was extremely useful when researching old recipes and ingredients. And I am very grateful to him for reading this manuscript and offering insightful comments and improvements, especially for pointing out that I'd transcribed one ingredient as *pounded finger* when (hopefully) I'd meant *pounded ginger*! The exceptional drawings and accompanying captions he has contributed have greatly enhanced the book.

Linne Matthews, my untiring, friendly editor at Pen and Sword, has worked with skill and dedication on all of my books and is always on hand to offer sage advice (and help with other herbs and spices as well).

To Caroline, my wife, fellow researcher and author: thank you for transcribing so many of the receipts in this book, designing the titles and for sharing your knowledge and your own research material. And of course, your stunning illustrations are extremely welcome additions to these chapters. On a personal note, you're such a modest, loving and generous soul that you will never come to realise how much of an indulgent, kind wife you are to me and what a wonderful mother you are to our two beautiful children, Lucy and Faye. The three of you inspire everything I do.

Picture Credits

Image 1, 3, 4 from author's archives.

Image 2 by kind permission of Archives cantonales vaudoises, Eb132/5 page 111.

Images 5, 6, 21, 22, 24, 25, 27, 28, 29, 30, 31, 32, 33, 34, 35 by Wellcome Collection, London. Copyrighted work available under Creative Commons Attribution only licence CC BY 4.0.

Images 7, 8, 9, 10, 11, 12, 13, 14, 15, 16, 17, 18, 19, 20, 23 by Peter Brears.

Image 26 is courtesy of the British Library www.bl.uk. No known copyright restrictions.

Front and back cover images and all titles and other illustrations by Caroline Rochford.

Preface

While researching my volume on Nostell Priory, the Palladian mansion in West Yorkshire, for the *Tales from the Big House* series (published in 2018 by Pen and Sword), I spent time at Wakefield History Centre viewing documents from the vast Nostell Priory collection. Within this archive are two Georgian 'receipt books' containing hundreds of old recipes for food and drink, and also dozens of remedies for the ills of the day, afflicting both man and beast. Receipt books were popular among the elite at this time and these volumes were compiled by Dame Sabine Winn, the Swiss wife of the 5th Baronet of Nostell, Sir Rowland Winn.

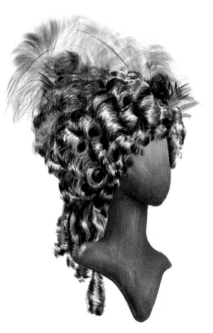

Sabine Louise May, née d'Hervart, was a 27-year-old widow from Vevey, Switzerland, when, on 4 December 1761, she married 22-year-old Rowland Winn, son of Nostell's fourth baronet, also called Rowland Winn. The younger Rowland had travelled to Vevey in August 1756 with his tutor, Isaac Dulon. He was studying in the country and was soon introduced to Madame May, with whom he instantly became infatuated. Unhappily married and not living with her husband, Sabine began an affair with the teenage heir, and when her husband, Gabriel May, died in 1759, the couple began making plans to marry.

2. The marriage of Sabine and Rowland at Vevey.

Sabine's father, Philip d'Hervart, a rich banker, did not approve of the match, nor did Sir Rowland, 4th Baronet, when news of his son's engagement reached him back in England. He swiftly wrote to his son to insist he chose 'a proper wife in your own country', listing what he thought were very sound reasons to think again. But the pair could not be swayed and following their marriage they moved to Yorkshire, living first at Badsworth (a location Sabine detested), and then, after the death of the 4th Baronet in 1765, at Nostell itself. They also kept a house at 11 St James's Square, Westminster, where a portrait of the couple by Hugh Douglas Hamilton, showing them standing in their large library at Nostell, was displayed prominently to impress visitors.

Sabine was by accounts a striking woman, described by a cousin of her husband's, Catherine Cappe, née Harrison, as possessing 'fine dark eyes sparkling with a radiance exclusively their own'. Cappe, writing in her memoirs, published in 1822 as *Memoirs of the life of the late Mrs Catharine Cappe, written by herself*, described Sabine as 'very beautiful' with a captivating manner and a 'great deal of vivacity'. She recalled first seeing her cousin's new bride:

When I first saw her, she was habited in a close vestment of pink satin, the colour not more delicate than her own fine complexion;

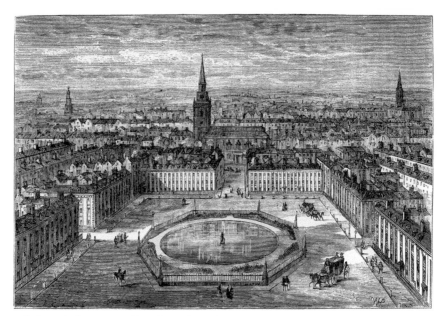

3. St James's Square in 1773, from Cassell's *Old and New London, volume four.*

she was tripping lightly along one of the great staircases; and seeing a stranger with one of the ladies of the family, ran up, and accosted us in French, with all the gaiety, ease, and politeness, peculiar to that nation [though of course Sabine was Swiss].

Catherine spent time as a guest of Sabine and Rowland, and as she got to know her cousin's wife better she grew to dislike her. She was alarmed by the 'irregular' hours kept by the couple, who were so lazy as to not sit down for breakfast until 'twelve or one', and didn't dine until 'seven or eight'. But what shocked her most was the way the couple treated an old lady who they'd also invited to stay with them. Catherine explained that the lady was not blessed with great judgement, and had in her youth been considered quite a beauty, and was thus somewhat vain and eager to please the couple. Apparently the new baronet possessed an odd-sounding 'electrical machine' with which he carried out 'experiments' and the poor elderly house guest was 'frequently the subject'. The Baronet also had an air pump into which he put small creatures, such as mice, to examine the effects of depriving them of oxygen. He knew the old dear detested mice, and playing on her fears he repeated threats to set them loose. When she wasn't being terrorised by the promise of having rodents run about her feet, Sabine was forcing the woman to stay up until the early hours of the morning, which, Catherine tells us, was ultimately 'ruinous to her health'. She decided to challenge Lady Winn about this and received the following reply: 'I keep her out of charity, and have a right to expect that she should conform to my pleasure.'

Sabine came to find life in England very difficult. Her husband was politically ambitious but never achieved his dream of becoming a Member of Parliament, except for a very brief period in 1768 when he

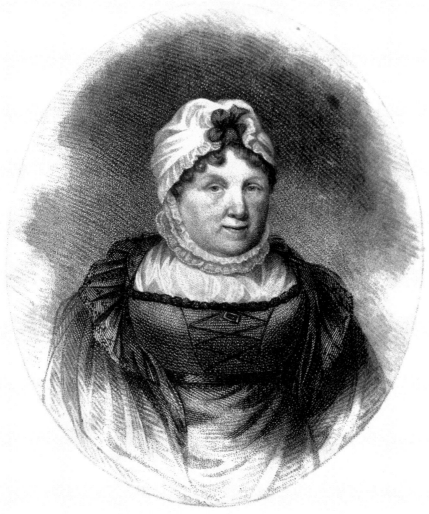

4. Catherine Cappe, from her memoirs.

conspired to win the seat in Pontefract by sending a mob of heavies to the town on the day of the election to beat up the supporters of his rivals, preventing them from casting their votes. He duly won the seat but the election was quickly declared void and he was rather less successful when it was rerun. In pursuit of high office, Sir Rowland travelled regularly and extensively, leaving Sabine alone and isolated at Nostell, especially following the death of her parents, with whom she had corresponded. On occassion, Sir Rowland left Sabine with little money to pay bills, for which she once admonished him in a letter, which was translated and included in Julie Day's 2008 book, *Elite Women's Household Management: Yorkshire, 1680–1810*. In the letter, Sabine tells her husband she was 'really very much vexed', asking him, 'what can I do? You should it seems to me, always leave a little money, at least when you are absent.' The couple also fell out with Sir Rowland's close family, not least his sisters, who accused him of withholding their inheritances, and few visitors were received at the big house.

In her book, Julie Day cited a translated copy of a letter Sabine received from her mother back in 1763 when the newly married couple were living at Badsworth. Mrs d'Hervart expressed her sorrow upon learning that her daughter had been putting on weight and suggested she take some exercise. Sabine's mother also recommended that she familiarised herself with the 'accounts of the house ... so as not to be a complete novice', explaining that this was what 'women are called on to do, and it is their duty, unless they want to be ruled over by their servants, instead of ruling over them'.

Julie Day did not find any evidence that Sabine ever took up her mother's advice about managing the accounts of the households she lived in (Badsworth, followed by Nostell), but there does exist a detailed inventory of the kitchen equipment at Nostell from Sabine's time as lady of the house. It is written in Sabine's native French, so was probably compiled by a lady's maid brought by Sabine from Switzerland to Nostell, or even by Sabine herself. It bears the date 9 February 1774. This document can be found in the Nostell Priory archives at Wakefield and has been translated for this book by Peter Brears. Entries from it include:

18 soup dishes
54 dishes with coats of arms
24 dishes without coats of arms
26 plates of different sizes
3 soup plates
5 fish plates
2 double dishes
1 double plate
10 large plates
3 small plates
15 plates, large and small
63 old dishes
2 soup basins
1 large dish
1 hand washing basin
7 egg cups
4 iron pots
2 candlesticks
2 saucepans

2 skimmers
3 gridrions
3 roasting spits
2 jack chains
3 little spits
1 coffee mill
2 waffle irons
1 platewarmer
10 pie dishes, large and small
2 cauldrons
An alembic [for distilling]
A coffee roaster
A basin for the servants' soup
2 mortars with a pestle
6 cafetières
5 chocolate pots
6 lanterns for the house
A night lantern and a lamp

It was around this time that Sabine developed a passion for collecting and compiling 'receipts' and two books into which she put some of these display a remarkably wide range of recipes and remedies. A loose paper, not found in either of the books but thought to have been written by Sabine, shows a remedy for 'L'alopocie', otherwise, alopecia. This required 2 ounces of cinnamon, 6 drams of cloves, an ounce and a half of lemon peel, an ounce of leaves from a red rose, 6 ounces of watercress, half a pound of scurvy grass and 3 pints of 'spirits of wine'. This last ingredient, more commonly called aqua vita, i.e. water of life, was understood in England to mean repeatedly distilled brandy. Once the ingredients had been sourced the maker of this remedy was instructed to:

Bruise the spices, cut the water cresses and scurvy grass small and macerate the whole in spirts of wine in a bottle well corked [for] the space of twenty four hours. Then distil to dryness in a vapour bath and afterwards rectify the distilled water by repeating the same process.

The method of application was not made clear. Was the potion meant to be consumed as a drink or massaged into the scalp?

Sabine's interest in simple, but practical, remedies was evident from the contents of a letter sent by Sir Rowland to John Murray, the London bookseller who had been based at 32 Fleet Street 'facing St Dunstan's Church' since 1762. In the letter, Mr Murray was told that 'Lady Wynn' was 'desirous to purchase a few books upon official botany' but was not sure which were 'the best and most esteemed modern works of that kind'. The letter continued:

> [Lady Winn] wishes to know what authors have writ upon these subjects in the clearest manner, upon the practical principals, and would be glad to be acquainted with the titles of such books and directions [on] how they are to be inquired for, not wishing to spend more time in pursuing the scientific knowledge of vegetables, [she] is desirous to be truly informed about the real virtues of simples, and proffers such authors as lay down plain and practical directions [on] how to prepare the best medicines from simples – [and] how they are to be taken and what is a proper dose.

Sir Rowland also requested some pages from the *Foreign Medical Review* journal, specifically those containing reviews of 'all the new books published on natural history, botany, materia medica, chemistry, anatomy, surgery, and the practice of physic in every part of the continent of Europe &c.' A reply sent on Murray's behalf suggested that *Lewis's List of Materia Medica; New Dispensatory* and *Pomets List of Drugs* 'will suit Lady Wynn'. Sir Rowland was also advised of forthcoming publications that had been 'printed for J. Murray No 32 Fleet Street'. These titles, presumably thought to be of interest to Sabine, included *Observations on Such Nutritive Vegetable as may be Substituted in the Place of Ordinary Food in Time of Scarcity* and *Farley's London Cookery, or the London Art of Cookery and Housekeepers Complete Assistant*. Another title Sabine must have had access to was called *The House-keeper's Pocket-Book*, printed in its fifth edition in 1751. This book contained a recipe for *A Regalia of Cucumbers*, which also appears in very similar wording in one of Sabine's own receipt books, right down to the number of cucumbers required to make it.

In her essay entitled *Between the Exotic and the Everyday: Sabine Winn at Home 1765–1798*, which appears in *A Taste for Luxury in Early Modern Europe* (published by Bloomsbury in 2017), Dr Kerry Bristol reveals some of Sabine's favourite purveyors of foodstuffs. She explains that whilst Sabine was able to source much of what she needed from Nostell's own estates, or from local dealers, she had to order better quality imports from London suppliers, such as:

Clarke and Pickering; Joseph Baker; Henry Pressey, a grocer of Nos 3 and 4 Henrietta Street, Covent Garden, who sold everything from coffee to candles, starch and mustard; and Joshua Long, grocer and tea dealer of No. 73 Cheapside, who supplied candied ginger and almonds in 1776 and white wine vinegar and Syrup de Capalain in 1785.

It was during 1785 when Sir Rowland died. In February of that year he was involved in a coach accident at Retford in Nottinghamshire while on one of his journeys to London. He left two children: a daughter, Esther Sabine, aged 16, and a 10-year-old son, also called Rowland, who became the 6th Baronet. Sabine was fiercely protective of her son, but she had a challenging relationship with Esther and never spoke to her again following the younger woman's elopement to Manchester with a lowly baker called John Williamson. Sabine took revenge on her daughter when writing her will. She disinherited Esther and also deprived her of an inheritence left to her by Sabine's own mother, leaving this instead to her son. Sabine made her reasons for doing so very clear in her will, which was proved in 1798:

And whereas my said daughter hath married very imprudently and entirely against the liking and will of me her mother ... by virtue of every other right power and authority vested in me I do hereby deprive her of the benefit ... and do give devise and bequeath the same and also all other my real and personal estate whatsoever and wheresoever and of what nature or kindsoever both in England and Switzerland or elsewhere subject nevertheless and charged and chargeable with the payment of all my just debts unto my dear son Sir Rowland Winn Baronet his heirs executors and administrators to hold and to the use of him my said son his heirs executors administrators and assigns forever.

As it happened, Sabine's son, the 6th Baronet, died unmarried and childless. Ironically, because he lacked an heir, Esther's own sons inherited Nostell, though not the baronetcy, which went to a cousin. Esther's sons duly changed their surnames from Williamson to Winn, and the youngest son, Charles, is the direct ancestor of the current Baron St Oswald, Charles Rowland Andrew Winn.

Less than two years after Sir Rowland's death, Sabine's name appeared in a curious notice in the *Leeds Intelligencer* newspaper, dated 12 December 1786. The notice comprised an advert for lectures that were to be performed in Leeds by Dr Katterfelto, a conjurer and experimental philosopher from Prussia who toured Britain from 1776 until his death in 1799. He was an odd fellow who performed with a black cat and 'two little black boys' and boasted the catchphrase 'Wonders! Wonders! Wonders!'

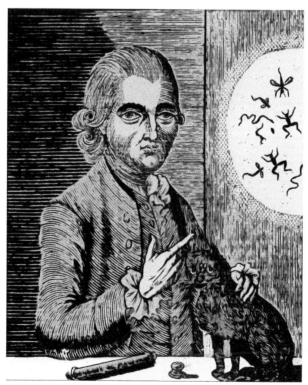

5. Dr Katterfelto with his black cat. *Country House Reader*, a blog by historian Julie Day, contains useful details about Dr Katterfelto's visit to Nostell Priory.

The doctor had made the bold, but untrue, claim that he'd ascended in a hot air balloon some fifteen years before Joseph-Michael and Jacques-Etienne Montgolfier had made their famous inaugural flight in 1783. It seems Katterfelto's services were in demand, though, for the Leeds newspaper notice also read: 'He is sorry he could not deliver his first lecture on the 4th Dec. last, being engaged for 5 nights at Lady Winn's at Nostell.' In fact, one of the remedies that follows, for curing madness in a dog, involves writing out a charm, or incantation, on a piece of buttered paper, which the mad dog was to be given to eat. '*Pega pega Effema, Pega pega Effema, Far Far Nar Nar, Nar Nar far far*', so went the charm – perhaps taught to Sabine by Dr Katterfelto himself during his stay.

The Nostell visit came at the height of Katterfelto's fame. It was during this period that he'd attracted the attention of the royal family, and according to various newspaper reports, he'd preformed for them at Buckingham House. Sabine had obviously fallen under his spell, too, affording him the best part of a week to demonstrate his skills. Less than five years later, Katterfelto would have given anything for such palatial accommodation if the following report, which appeared in the provincial press, is anything to go by:

On Wednesday last the celebrated Dr Katterfelto, (M.D. and F.R.S.) was committed to the House of Correction at Kendal, as a rogue and vagabond; and was also convicted of profane cursing and swearing, (very unseemly indeed for a *divine* and *moral* philosopher) and paid the penalty inflicted by law for this offence. He had been previously informed by the Magistrates that he would not be permitted to perform his 'juggling tricks' in the town: but placing too strong a reliance on the *magic* powers of his *Morocco Black Cat*, the Doctor disregarded the official warning, and so incurred the punishment and the disgrace.

Towards the end of her life, Sabine became unwell with rheumatic gout. According to a family doctor, she 'become very stout and was wheeled about in a quaint big wheeled chair', and had to use poles to exercise. Sabine died in September 1798, leaving her bitter will, the full story of which can be read in *Tales From the Big House: Nostell Priory*. In that

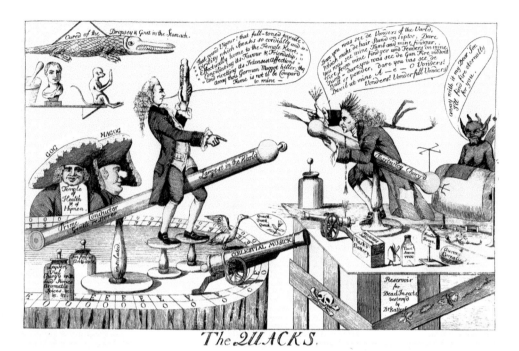

6. 'The Quacks', an etching printed by W. Humphrey in 1783 showing Katterfelto and another quack, called Graham, in battle.

book can also be found a sample of sixteen of Sabine Winn's recipes and remedies. A fuller selection appears in the pages that follow.

I consulted many documents held at the National Archives in Kew when writing my earlier book about Nostell Priory. And following a productive day there, my wife Caroline and I ventured into the capital and paid a customary visit to the antiquarian bookshops on Charing Cross Road. In one of these we were lucky enough to stumble across a large, leatherbound tome with intricate gilding on the spine and the edges of its 600 pages. After a bit of good old Yorkshire bartering we were delighted to be able to take it home with us to Wakefield. This treasured find is simply titled *Receipt Book* and dates back to 1807. In the book's introduction, the unnamed author explained that he had inherited a large collection of *'receipts in cookery, medicine, etc, which had descended, as an heirloom, through several successive generations'*. Having sampled some of the hints and tips for himself, he found them to be of great value and set about expanding his collection by consulting every relevant book or manuscript he could get his hands on. He sought the help of family, friends, *'intelligent travellers and highly respectable characters'*, inviting them to submit their own failsafe receipts. For two decades he worked on his collection until he finally had enough material to publish his book, which, he claimed, was *'absolutely without a parallel in any part of the world'*. Not seeking to play down his work, he selected a somewhat grandiose subtitle, and I hope readers will forgive me for citing it below in all its glory:

A Universal Repository of Useful Knowledge and Experience in all the various Branches of Domestic Economy, including Scarce, Curious and Valuable SELECT RECEIPTS and CHOICE SECRETS in cookery, medicine, confectionary, pastry, brewing, distilling, pickling, preserving, perfumery, dyeing, gilding, painting, varnishing, agriculture, farriery, gardening, hunting, fishing, fowling, etc, etc, etc, with specifications of approved patent medicines; all the most serviceable preparations for Domestic Purposes; and numerous successful Improvements in the Ornamental as well as Useful Arts, Manufactures, etc, extracted from the Records of the Patent Office; and translated from foreign books and journals, in all the languages of Europe, the whole forming a Complete Library of Valuable Domestic Knowledge, and General Economy; selected from the Experience of Ages, and combined with all the chief Modern Discoveries and Improvements of our own and other Countries, in those Useful and Elegant Arts which not only contribute to Happiness, the Convenience, and the Comfort of Civilised and Social Life, but even to the Preservation and Prolongation of Life itself

As our author was a Georgian, many of his collected receipts may have been known to Sabine's generation, and perhaps even Sabine herself; thus a selection from this intriguing volume has been included in my book. These focus on health and medicine and therefore appear in the remedies section. I have edited some of these to make them a little more readable. They are marked under their titles '1807' or '1815' (the year in which the author published a second edition) so a reader can tell these and Sabine's remedies apart.

A Note on the Nostell Priory Source Material

In Sabine's original receipt books each receipt is presented as a stream of prose with the ingredients and methods unseparated. So that a modern reader can follow, and hopfully try, some of the receipts, I have presented the ingredients and methods separately. To that end, I have modernised the spellings and measurements of the ingredients but mostly retained original spellings for the methods, except where this renders the text confusing or difficult to read, such as when a word like *flower* is used when *flour* is meant and *pair* when *pare* is intended. In these cases, today's spellings have been used. Grammer and punctuation is somewhat lacking in Sabine's receipts and therefore this has been added where appropriate. Titles have been altered here and there.

Occasionally, exact measurements were not given in Sabine's books. For example, some receipts simply state 'a spoonful' without explaining the size of the spoon required. According to food historian Peter Brears, the spoons used in cooking around this time were equivalent in size to modern dessert spoons, though some receipts do specify that a tablespoon ought to be used. The term quart is often used and this has been expressed in the modern ingredients as two imperial UK pints, but I have left the word quart in the methods. Pound becomes lb and ounce oz but again, the original words are retained in the methods. Temperatures are not expressed in the original receipts beyond phrases like 'a very soft oven', 'a quick oven', 'a warm oven' etc. and timings are sometimes omitted entirely. So speaking from personal experience, a little trial and error, and a dash of common sense will be required!

Please use caution if attempting any of these receipts. Many of the recipes will work really well, offering very flavoursome dishes, but some are included purely for interest alone. Take the recipe for *Pretty Cream*: this required five or six drops of ambergris; you'll need to kill a whale to obtain this ingredient. And many of the remedies, written before the dawn of modern science, are obviously dangerous and should not be attempted under any circumstances. Take as another example, *Water for the Eyes*, which directs you to add *tutty* to the mixture. This is a substance obtained from the flues of zinc smelting furnances, consting of zinc oxide! This receipt claims to have restored sight to the blind, but will probably remove this sense from the seeing if *tutty* is rubbed in the eyes. The same applies to *calamine*, sold today as a lotion that dries very quickly on the skin and is usually used to relieve itching from bites and diseases such as chicken pox and crucially comes with a warning that it should not be applied to the eyes. In Sabine's receipt books, this forms part of a remedy for another eye wash. A remedy to stop you feeling sick suggests taking thirty drops of liquid laudanum – as a Class A substance under the Misuse of Drugs Act 1971, it's probably best you don't. And it's not likely any of your pet pooches will appreciate being force-fed the charm on buttered paper, previously described.

If the original receipt books are of further interest, they can be found in the Nostell Priory archive at Wakefield History Centre under the references WYW1352/3/4/7/3 and WYW1352/3/4/7/5.

Recipes

Cakes, Biscuits and Bread

Apricot Cakes for Winter
Barberry Wafers
The Cake that will keep Half a
   Year
Caraway Cake
Clear Apriot Cakes
Currant Cakes
Diet Bread
Donuts
The Duchess of York's Cake
Dutch Wafers
French Bread
Gingerbread
Another Gingerbread
Mrs Wyatt's Gingerbread
How to Ice Cakes
K. Winn's Ratafia Biscuits
Lady Lawley's Cheesecakes
Lady Westmoreland's Little
   Cakes
Lemon Cakes
Mrs Hunter's Cake
Mrs Oliver's Cheesecakes
Mrs Waterton's Orange Cakes
Nuns' Biscuit
Orange Biscuits
Orange Cheesecake

Paris Royal Biscuits
Plum Cake
Mrs Rooke's Very Good Plum
   Cake
Savoy Biscuits
A Seed Cake
Another Seed Cake
Shortcakes
Spanish Biscuits
Wafers
Wiggs

Cheeses, Custards and Creams

Almond Cream
Apricot Custard
Barley Cream
Custard
Egg Cheese
To Make Fresh Cheese
Lady Harbord's Marigold Cheese
Mrs Drake's Sack Posset
Mrs Eall's Custard
Mrs Spencer's Lemon Cream
Orange Cream
Pretty Cream
Ramekins
Scottish Cream
Tea Cream

Jams, Jellies, Pickles and Preserves

Green Apple Preserve
Green Plum Preserve
India Pickles
Mrs Fortescue's Gooseberries
Mrs Winn's Pickled Mushroom
Orange and Lemon Marmalade
Pickled Artichokes
Pickled Button Mushrooms
Pickled Cabbage
Pickled Cucumbers
Pickled Indian Pepper
Pippin Marmalade
Preserve Gooseberries as Green
   as they Grow
A Way to Preserve Green Pippins
Preserve Oranges
Preserve Peascods
Ripe Plums
Sir Theodore Colladon's Peach
   Flower Syrup
The Very Old Recipe for
   Raspberry Jelly
The Very Old Way of Preserving
   Cherries
Walnut Ketchup
White Quince Marmalade

Meat, Fish and Poultry

Bake a Leg of Mutton
Buttered Chicken
Creamy Chicken Pie
Galantine of Rabbits
How to Roast a Rump of Beef
Meat Patties
Mother's Scotch Collops

Mrs Eall's Mumbled Hare
Mrs Thornhill's Chicken Fricassee
Mutton Rumps
Oyster Loaves
Oyster Pie
Pickled Westphalia Ham
Pork Sausages
Potted Hare
Potted Lobster
Roast Duck
Stew a Calf's Head
Stewed Carp
Stewed Haddock or Perch
Stewed Pigeons with Cabbage
The Duchess of Portsmouth's
   Stewed Beef
Turkey à la Daube
Very Good Wood-Smoked Hams

Puddings, Pies and Sweets

Barberry Comfits
Batter Pudding
Beef Pie in Blood
Candy Flowers
Champagne Gooseberries
Christmas Pyes
Clear Apple Fritters
Excellent White Puddings
Flummery
Fritters
Grandma Layer's Very Good
   Black Puddings
Green Pudding
Ice Cream
Lady St Quintin's Dutch
   Pudding
Lady Winn's Mother's Fritters

Little Baked Puddings
To Make a Pudding
Marrow Pudding
Mince Pies
Mrs Cook's Almond Pudding
Mrs Cook's Liver Pudding
Mrs Cook's Oatmeal Pudding
Mrs Eall's Candied Cowslips
Mrs Eall's Goosberry Fool
Mrs Wiseman's Pancakes
New College Pudding
Orange Tarts
Rice Pudding
Sago Pudding
Snow Balls
Spanish Pap
Sugar of Red Roses
Tansy Pudding
White Puddings

Soups, Sauces and Sides
Artichoke Florentine
Cauliflower au Galantine
Dressing for an English Turtle
    (Mock Turtle)
Fish Sauce
French Beans with Cream
How to Prepare Asparagus
Morels à la Crème
Mrs K. Winn's Onion Soup
Mustard
Pistachio Cream for Chicken
Regalia of Cucumbers
Soup

Wines, Spirits, Vinegars and Waters
Boxed Wine
Cherry Wine
Cinnamon Water
Cowslip Wine
Duchess of Norfolk's Punch
Elder Wine
Elderflower Vinegar
Elderflower Wine
Gooseberry Wine
Lady Strickland's Strong Mead
Lady Sunderland's Elder Water
Lady Winn's Mother's
    Gooseberry Wine
Lemon Brandy
Liquorice Juice
Mrs Eall's Mead
Orange Wine
Another Orange Wine
Quince Wine
Raspberry Brandy
Right Red Dutch Currant Wine
Sage Wine
Shrub
Sir Rowland's Milk Water
Strong Mead
Sycamore wine
Usquebaugh
Vinegar

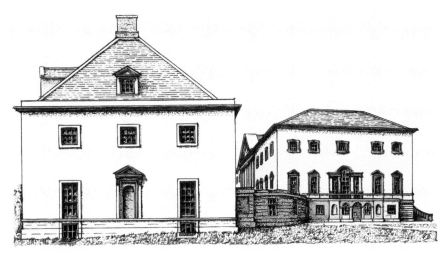

7. Exterior of Nostell Priory kitchen by Peter Brears. Designed in the early 1730s, the north-western pavilion of Nostell Priory incorporated a bakehouse in the basement, a full-height kitchen and a scullery on the ground floor, and servants' bedrooms in the first floor and attic.

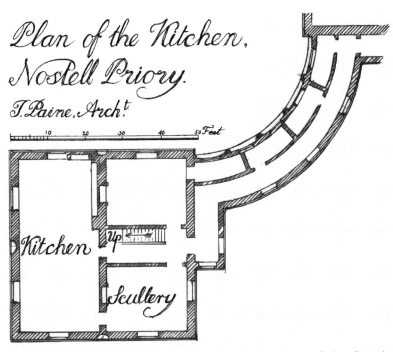

8. Plan of Nostell Priory kitchen by Peter Brears based on that in Colen Campbell's *Vitruvius Britannicus*. In order to protect the house from the noise, smells and fire risk of the kitchen, their only link was a pair of curving corridors at ground level, and another below to connect the cellars.

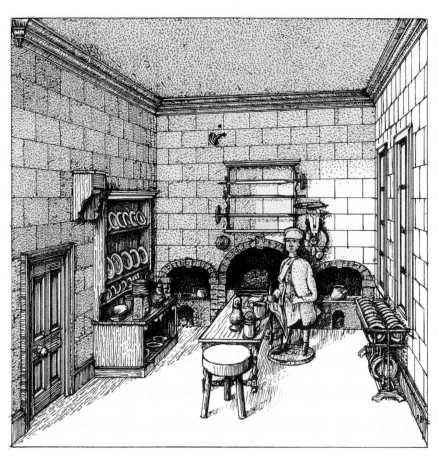

9. Drawing by Peter Brears showing the kitchen from the famous Dolls' House at Nostell, designed in about 1740 under the direction of Lady Winn and often erroneously attributed to Thomas Chippendale. See *Tales From the Big House: Nostell Priory* by the present writer for a brief account of the Dolls' House. This fine kitchen in miniature has a typical three-arched arrangement of a roasting range flanked by a pair of charcoal stoves. Other features include a towel roller, a dresser, a spit rack and clockwork jack over the fire, a chopping block and a fine dish-rack.

Cakes, Biscuits and Bread

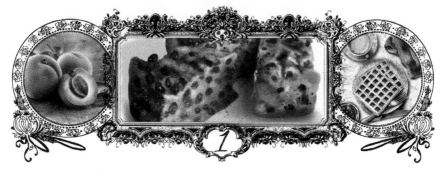

1

abine's receipt books contain a large number of entries for sweet cakes, many of which are made with fruits such as apricot, lemon and orange. Also popular in her books are recipes for gingerbread. Peter Brears explains in *Gentlewoman's Kitchen: Great Food in Yorkshire, 1650–1750* that from the beginning of the eighteenth century, the town of Wakefield, which is a short distance from Nostell Priory, was renowned for its gingerbread.

A receipt contributed by one of the Winn family is *K. Winn's Ratafia Biscuits*. This biscuit took its name from a liqueur similarly flavoured with almond, apricot, cherry or peach kernels. It closely resembles recipies from early eighteenth-century cookbooks, perhaps tweaked a little by K. Winn, who was probably Sabine's sister-in-law, the spinster Katherine Winn.

Other highlights include *Nuns' Biscuit*, and recipes supplied by Ladies Lawley and Westmoreland for *Little Cakes* and *Cheesecakes*, respectively. This section also includes breads in the form of *Diet Bread*, which in this case was sweet bread flavoured with caraway seeds and lemon peel, and, perhaps due to Sabine's European influence, *French Bread*, and also *Dutch Wafers*.

The final receipt in this section is for *Wiggs*. These are small cakes, what we might call buns, made to a simple recipe of flour, butter, sugar, milk and yeast, which were formerly served at funerals in the north of

England. Ivan Day of Historic Food, based in Cumbria, cites an account of the funeral expenses of a woman from the Lake District who died in 1728. This shows that Wiggs were provided to the mourners, and cost her widower 7 shillings for '14 dozen at 14 to the Dozen'.

Apricot Cakes for Winter

Ingredients:

1lb of apricots
1lb of double refined sugar
Glass jars, for storage

Method: Take one pound of Apricoks indifferent ripe, pare them and quarter them then take one pound of the best double refind sugar take halfe of it & boyle it to a candy then put in your apricok & boyle them a pretty while then take your other halfe pound of sugar finely beaten & put to them & then boyle them a pace 'till they come to be thick then glass them up for winter. Keep them pretty warm but not too hott when you turn them outt.

Barberry Wafers

Ingredients:

Barberry pulp (as prepared when making Barberry Comfits) [*see page* 73]
Caster sugar
Sheets of baking paper

Method: Take your Pulp prepared as before [for Barberry Comfits], then put to it as much of the Sugar as you think will be Sufficient to make Dry, then take about 3 or 4 Spoonfulls in a Silver Ladle and hold itt over a Stove till tis very Hott butt if it Eather Boyles or Simers itt will never Dry. Then spred em upon Papers the size you would have em then in half an hour you may role 'em up into Little round Drops. These are to be heated in the same manner and then Dropt upon paper. The paper must be Sliced and when the wafers are Dry enough to take off the papers you must wett the papers a Little.

The Cake that will keep Half a Year

Ingredients:

5lb of fine flour
6lb of currants
½lb of sugar
⅓oz of mace
⅓oz of an ounce of cloves
⅓oz of nutmeg
6 eggs
16 yolks
½ pint of orange flower water
1 pint of the best ale yeast
2½ pints of butter
1½ pints of cream
¼lb of candied orange, lemon and citron peel

Method: Take 5 pd of fine Flour dry'd well in an Oven, 6 pd of Currance, half a pd of Sug'r, of mace, cloves & nutmegs, an Ounce together. Beat 22 eggs with half a pint of orange flower water, take out 16 whites, then take your Sug'r & Spice beaten very small, mix it with your Flour, then take a pint of the best Ale yest & rub it into your Flour, then put in your eggs & 2 po'd & a half of Butter melted in a pint & half of Cream, but be sure your Cream does not boyle & when it is but blood warm put it to the Flour, & stir it well together & set it by the Fire to rise an hour then take it up & put in the Currance & shred a quart'r of a p'd of Canded Orange, Lemmon & Citron-peal, & set it in a quick Oven. An hour will bake it. Make your Cake lowest in the middle a little it will be even when baked.

Caraway Cake

Ingredients:

4 pints of fine flour
6 spoonsful of good ale yeast
Cream
1lb of sweet butter
1lb of caraway comfits, plus extra for decoration

Method: Take 2 quarts of fine Flour, put to it 6 spoonfulls of good ale yest & wet it with cream. Knead it stiff as you do White-bread, then set it to rise at the Fire, & take a pound of Sweet butter & a pound of Carroway Comfitts & work 'em together into the paste between your hands & make it lightly up into a Cake. Strew a few of the Comfits on the top, set in the Oven, not too hot. Stop the Mouth of the Oven that it may rise. You may try the Oven for heat by putting a piece of Paper in it. If it does not burn the paper, it is of a due heat.

Clear Apricot Cakes

Ingredients:

Apricots
Sugar (equal to the weight of the apricot juice)

Method: Pare your apricoks & put them in a deep Earthen pott, & set it in a skillet of wat'r to boile half an hour, then poor itt into a tiffany sive, for the clear to run from itt. Take the weight of the Juice in the best Sug'r, boil it to a candie, then put in the Juice. Put it in clear cake glasses & dry it in a stove. The thick pulp you may use just so for cakes, call'd past of apricoks.

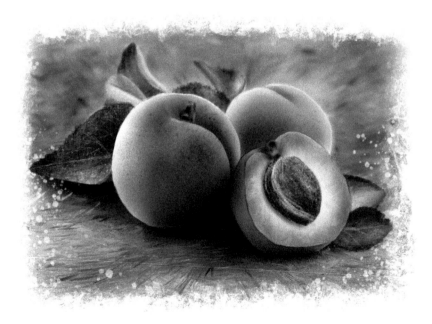

Currant Cakes

Ingredients:

2lb of flour
½lb of sugar
4 yolks
2 egg whites
½lb of butter
Rose water
6 spoonsful of warmed cream
2lb of currants

Method: Take 2 pound of flower dry'd in the oven, halfe a pound of sugar, finely beaten 4 yolks and 2 whites of Eggs, half pound of Buter washed in Rose water, 6 spoonfulls of Cream warmed then take 2 pound of Currance wash very well. So mix them all to gether make 6 or 8 cakes of it the past is very light so that you must flower your hand well for that you must take a Lump & cut it keeping them round they will take a pretty while to bake & will not be good to eat till they be 2 days old. They will keep a Great while.

Diet Bread

Ingredients:

1lb of double refined sugar
8 eggs
13oz of flour
½oz of caraway seeds, or the peel of 1 lemon

Method: Take a pound of double refin'd Sugar, finely Beat & Sifted, 8 Eggs, yolks & whites beat w'th a whisk half an Hour or more. Put the Sugar into it by degrees as you beat 'em and 13 oz of Flour dry'd & Sifted. Put it in a little at a time w'th half an oz of caraway seeds. If you like the tast of Lemon you must Grate the peall & put in, instead of the seeds. Beat all well together. Half an Hour will Bake it.

Donuts

Ingredients:

¼ of a peck of flour
2 spoonsful of yeast
1 egg
½lb of butter
Sugar, to taste
Spices, to taste
Currants, to taste (optional)
Hog's lard

Method: Take a quart'r of a peck of flour, 2 spoonfulls of yest & 1 egg. Put in half a p'd of Butter or more into boyleing water to work it up into a light paste. Put in Sug'r & Spice as you think fit. You may put in Currance if you please. So make 'em up into nuts & boyle 'em in Hogs Lard.

The Duchess of York's Cake

Ingredients:

1lb of white sugar
1lb of melted fresh butter, plus extra for greasing
12 eggs
2 yolks
1 spoonful of rose water
3 spoonsful of Canary sack (otherwise fortified wine)
½ a spoonful of cloves, mace and nutmeg, crushed and mixed
    together
1½lb of flour and currants
Fine sugar

Method: Take a p'd of white Sug'r, beat it, then mingle the Sug'r with a p'd of fresh Butter melted, 14 eggs (2 whites left out) a spoonful of Rose water, 3 of Canary, half a Spoonfull of Cloves, mace & nutmeg beaten together, then put to it a pound & half of Flour & Currants, then butter papers & drop 'em on w'th a Spoon wetted with fair water, then bind 'em with papers of the bignesse you would have 'em. When you have set 'em in the Oven, sift fine Sug'r on 'em.

Dutch Wafers

Ingredients:

2lb of flour
1lb of fresh butter, plus extra for serving
3 pints of milk
½ a pint of cream
1 glass of sack (otherwise fortified wine)
5 eggs
5 yolks
4 Naples biscuits, crushed
½ spoonful of cinnamon, plus extra for sprinkling on top
2 spoonsful of yeast
½ a spoonful of salt
Sugar, sprinkled on top

Method: Take two pound of flour, one pound of Fresh butter, three pints of milk, half a pint of Creame, a glass of sack, tenn Eggs (five of them with oute the whites), four naples biskcaks, half a spoonfull of beaten sinnamon, two spoonfulls of yest, half a spoonfull of salt. If you do not bake it the same day then put in but one spoonfull of yest. When baked putt over them suggar and sinnamon and a little butter if you please.

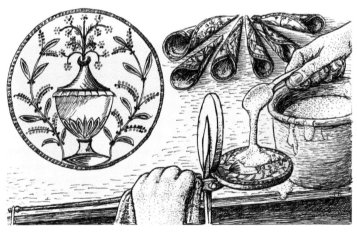

10. Wafers by Peter Brears. Wafers were made by pouring batter into a pair of engraved wafer-tongs that had been heated over a charcoal stove. Once clamped together, the irons rapidly cooked the batter, meanwhile sending out squeaking jets of steam. After, the wafers were removed, rolled into shape and left to cool to crispness.

French Bread

Ingredients:

½ a peck of flour, plus extra for dusting
Six eggs
1 pint of cream
3 pints of new milk
Salt, to taste

Method: Take half a peck of flour, 6 Eggs, a pint of Cream, 3 pints of new milk and a little salt. Beat all these together with your hand 'till they are well mixed, then have Dishes well floured and put the Dough in. So let it stand a quarter of an hour to harden, then put it in the Oven. It must be pretty hott.

Gingerbread

Ingredients:

3lb of fine flour
1 pint of honey
1lb of sugar
A little sack [sherry, or fortified wine]
Ginger
Coriander
Caraway seeds
Candied lemon and citron peel
Butter for greasing your pans

Method: To three pound of fine flour take one pint of honey, one pound of white sugar, make 'em boyle and scum it clean. Let it stand a little and put in a little sack to the honey and sugar then stir it into the flour. Put in your ginger, coriander and what caraway seeds you please, beaten and sifted and add some slices of candied lemon and citron peel and caraway comfits. And when 'tis mingled set it against the fire to rise 'till your oven is hot. Butter your pans very little and if they are not a little buttered they will not come out. Set 'em in a quick oven – about an hour will bake 'em.

Another Gingerbread

Ingredients:

2 pounds of sugar
½ a pint of milk
1lb of butter
2oz of ginger
1oz of a mixture of spices:
    Nutmeg
    Mace
    Cloves
    Galangal
    Cardamom seeds
    Long pepper
    Coriander seed (optional)
Flour (enough to make a dough)

Method: Take 2 pound of Sugar, put to it half a pint of Milk & a pound of Butter. Set 'em over the fire, let it be no hotter than just to melt the Butter. To 2 pound of sugar you must put 2 ounces of Ginger & an Ounce of other Spice: Nutmegs, mace & cloves, Galingale, Cardamon seeds, Long-pepper, & if you please, a little Coriander seed. Put all your Spice into your flour, & make it up into a Stiff past, & roll it as you please.

Mrs Wyatt's Gingerbread

Ingredients:

3 pounds of treacle
1½lb of butter, plus extra for greasing
1lb and 2oz of sugar
1½oz of beaten ginger
1 large nutmeg
Peel of 3 three fresh lemons
4½lb of flour
Peel of citrons and oranges, to taste

Method: Take Three Pound of Treakle, one pound and a half of Butter, one Pound two Ounces of Sugar, one Ounce & a half of beat Ginger, one Large nutmeg, the Peel of Three fresh Lemmons, shred very fine. Melt the Butter to Oyle, & put all the other Ingrediants to it. Make it scalding hot, mix it well, let it stand till almost cold, then put four pound and a half of Flour, and as much Cittron and Orange peel as you think fit. Put the Cakes on Tin plates, Butter'd, and Bake them in a Slow Oven.

How to Ice Cakes

Ingredients:

1½lb of double refined sugar
5 egg whites
2 spoonsful of rosewater
Homemade cake

Method: Take a pound & a halfe of Duble Refind Sugar beaten & strained through the finest sieve you can gett. Put into it the whites of 5 Eggs & 2 spoon full of rosewater. Keep it a beating all the time your cake is a bakeing which will be about 2 hours then draw your cake forth out the oven & pick your dry'd currance off [the top of the cake] & spread the Icing very smooth all over and set it a Little in the oven to dry but have a care you do not discolour itt.

K. Winn's Ratafia Biscuits

Ingredients:

¼lb of bitter almonds, blanched and beaten
¼lb of sweet almonds, blanched and beaten
2 or 3 spoonsful of orangeflower water
6 eggs
2 yolks
1lb of double refined sugar, plus extra for sprinkling
½ a pound of flour

Oven-safe card containers

Method: Take a quarter of a pound of Bitter Allmonds & as many sweet Allmonds, blanch't & beat very small in a marble morter with 2 or 3 sponfulls of orrangflower water. Then take eight Eggs, leave out 2 of the whites. Beat them very well & mix them with the Allmonds then take a pound of Dubble refin'd Shuger, fine sifted, & half a pound of flour well dry'd. Mix all these together in your morter & let them stand in it for half an hower, then put them in pans made of Cards & sift some Shuger over them. A quarter of an Hower will bake them.

Lady Lawley's Cheesecakes

Ingredients:

½ a pint of cream
¾lb of butter
¾lb of sugar
10 eggs
2 yolks
3 large lemons (the juice of one and the grated peel of all three)
Orange flower water, to taste

Method: Take half a pint of cream, three quarters of a pound of Butter, 3 quarters of a pound of Sugar, 12 Eggs, (leave out 2 of the whites), the peel of 3 Lemons grated, the juice of one if a large one. Mix these well together & set over a Jentle Fire & keep it stirring 'till it is thick then add a little Orange Flower water. This quantity will make 3 dozen of Small Chesecakes. A Quick oven: half an houre will bake them.

Lady Westmoreland's Little Cakes

Ingredients:

1lb of flour
1lb of unsalted butter
Orange flower water or rose water, to wash the butter in, plus 1
    spoonful of orange flower water
4 or 5 yolks
A few caraway seeds
Sugar, to taste
Fine sugar, for dusting

A drinking glass, for cutting round the cakes

Method: Take a pound of flour and as much butter, unsalted, and well washed in orange flower water or Rose water, 4 or 5 yolks of Eggs, a few Carryway seeds, a spown full of Orange flower water and a little Shugar. Break the Butter into the flower very small and make it into past. Handle it as little as you can. Role it out and cut it with Glass into Little Cakes. Put them upon Tinns or paper. Sift some fine suger over them & put them into an oven not too hott.

Lemon Cakes

Ingredients:

Double refined caster sugar
Lemon juice (or, for violet cakes, orange flower water or rose water)
Violets (for violet cakes)

Method: Take Duble Refind sugar & sieve it very finely through a cane sieve then put it into a Skillet & set it over the fire & then wett it with your Juice of Lemon & let it be Pretty hott & all the Sugar dissolved. Then if you would have blister'd cakes drop as fast as you can upon papers and if you would not have them blister'd drop them upon plates. You may make violet cakes this way in stead of Lemon. You must wett your sugar with orange flower water or Rose water & let that boile a candy & then put in your violetts & so drop them as fast as you cann.

Mrs Hunter's Cake

Ingredients:

10 eggs
1lb of caster sugar
¾lb of flour
Butter, for greasing

Method: Take 10 Eggs. Beat them half an houer. Sieve a pound of fine Suger. Put it to your Eggs and beat them an houer Longer. Take 3 quarters of a pound of flour. Dry itt well. When it is Cold put it to your Eggs and Sugar, then beat it half an houer or more. Butter your tinn. It will take too Houers Baking!

Mrs Oliver's Cheesecakes

Ingredients:

The curd of 12 pints of new milk
4 pints of cream
15 yolks
1lb of currants
1¼lb of sugar
¼oz of mace
1lb of flour

Method: Take the Curd of six quarts of new milk & whey it well and beat it in a mortar. Then take two quarts of Creame, keeping a porringer full of the Cream to make the crust. Then take the yolks of twelve Eggs & boyle the eggs & creame together 'till they come to a tender curd & when it is cold mix your creame curd and your cheese curds together then put in a pound of currance and a pound of shugar and a quarter of an ounce of mace very well beaten. Take a pound of flour and the yolks of three Eggs and a quarter of a pound of shugar finely beaten & scarch then boyle your creame and coule it a little and so make it into a stiff past and beate it well w'th your rouleing pin and so roule it oute thin. This is the way to make the crust for the Cheese Cakes.

Mrs Waterton's Orange Cakes

Ingredients:

Oranges with thick rind (enough to make 1lb of prepared flesh
   and rind)
1⅛lb of double refined sugar

Method: Take the thickest rinded orinatges as you can gett. Cutt them in quarters & squese out all the Juse then pick all the meat from the skines & seeds. Put itt to your Juse then cutt the Rindes in thine pieces. Boyle them in Severall waters 'till the biterness is gon then tack them cleare from the water, cutt them small & put to the meat. Mix them well together. To a pound of these take a pound & halfe quartor of Duble refined Sugar. Boyle itt to a Suger againe then put in your orinatges. Lett itt stand over the fier for som time but not boyle. Then put it into Glasses. When it is canded of one side, turne them.

Nuns' Biscuit

Ingredients:

1lb of caster sugar
½lb of blanched almonds
5 or 6 egg whites
5 yolks
1 lemon peel, grated, or candied citron
¼lb of flour
Butter, for greasing
Fine sugar, for sprinkling

Biscuit pans

Method: Take a p'd of Loafe Sug'r sifted, half a p'd of blanch'd Almonds, beat 'em in a stone mortar very fine with 5 or 6 Whites of eggs new laid. Put your Sug'r into a deep broad Bason with the yolks of 5 eggs. When they are well mix'd together stir in the Almonds by degrees. Grate in the peal of a raw Lemmon or 2 & a little peice of candied Citron & let it all be stirr'd together a good while then stirr in a quart'r of a p'd of flour finely sifted & fill it into long Bisket pans ab't half full. Let your pan be well butter'd then set 'em in the Oven. Strew a little fine Sug'r on 'em. Bake 'em quickly, shutting up the oven as soon as they begin to colour a top, then turn 'em upon papers. Set 'em in the Oven again to harden the sides a little & then they are enough.

Orange Biscuits

Ingredients:

6 oranges
Sugar, the same weight (plus half) as the prepared oranges
Juice of one lemon

Method: Take 6 Orinages, cut them & take out the Juce & Seeds & boyle them in a kettle of water 'till they be very tender then when cold take off the outer rind & beat each of them small with piping water & when beaten small enough put in the weight and a halfe of fine sugar

& beat them together. Then wring in the Juice of one Lemon and then drop it up on Plates into the form of Round cakes as big as biskets & set them in a warm place or stove till they be fitt to turn.

Another method …

Ingredients:

1lb of orange peel
1½lb of sugar

Method: Take a pound of orinorges, a pound & a halfe of sugar. Lay them in water for eight dayes & shift them twice a day then boile them 'till they be tender in two severall waters but the last water is to be as hot as the first before you put them in. Then wipe them dry & take out the Juce & white skin & Leave only the peell and put a pound & a halfe of Sugar to a pound of that peell & beate it finely together in a morter. Then take it out & lay it thinn about an Inch thick upon a glass and dry it. Then cut it in quarters before it be dry.

Orange Cheesecake

Ingredients:

2 oranges
Juice of 1 lemon, plus extra, if desired
¼lb of butter
5 yolks
1½ egg whites
1lb of sugar
Puff pastry, for the base

Method: Note: Steepe in faire wotter a night before you put it in to lemons. Take 2 oranges and pare off the Yellow Rinde and Lay it in Steepe in Juce of one Lemmon all night. Then Beate them in a Stone Mortor and when they are veary fine putt to them a quarter of a pound of butter with the yolks of five eggs and the whites of one and a halfe, a pound of Shuger and the meate of The Oranges. Be sure to pick outt all the Seeds and Strings and if you think it nott sharpe enough add to it Juce of Lemmons. It will take an houre to beate it all together in the mortor and Soe putt them into Puff Paste.

Paris Royal Biscuits

Ingredients:

1lb of eggs
½lb of flour
Lemon peel, to taste
Sugar, to taste, plus extra for sifting
Butter, for greasing

Tins, for baking

Method: Take a pound of new laid Eggs in the Shell. Break them some time before you beate them. Beat the whites & yolks separate. Leave out two of the yolks. To the rest add half a pound flour well dryed and a Little fresh Lemon peel grated. Add the Sugar & the peel and beat the whites to a stiff Froath at the same time. When done add them & the Flour to the yolks & Sugar. Just mix them well together & fill your Tins rather above half full. Sift some fine Sugar over them. Put them in an oven. A little time will bake them. The tins must be very well Butter'd.

Plum Cake

Ingredients:

3½lb of the finest flour
The yolks of 12 eggs
2 pints of cream
1lb of butter
½lb of loafsugar
½oz of large mace
½ pint of the best ale
A little damask rose water
3½lb of currants

Method: Take 3 pound & a half of the finest flour, well dry'd, the yolkes of 12 well-beaten eggs, & a quart of boyl'd cream. Put a pound of butter to it, half a pound of loafe-sugar, mixed with your flour, half an ounce of large mace, half a pint of the best ale, & a little damask rose water. Make a round hole in the flour & put all these ingredients into it. Then strew some of the same flour into the hole, the thickness of half an inch. Then let it stand 'till it workes over, then mix it up & take 3 pound & a half of currants & put into it as you mix it. Clap it on a paper, well-butter'd with a hoop about it. Set it into the oven & let it stand an hour & 3 quarters.

Mrs Rooke's Very Good Plum Cake

Ingredients:

4lb of flour
8lb of currants
2lb of double refined sugar
1oz of shredded mace
½lb of citron
¼lb of candied orange
¼lb of candied lemon
4lb of butter
32 eggs
1 gill of sack, otherwise fortified wine

Method: The day before you intend to make your cake you must dry 4 pounds of flour but be carefull not to Brown it in the drying. Wash 8 pounds of Courans in 3 different waters but don't let them lye in the

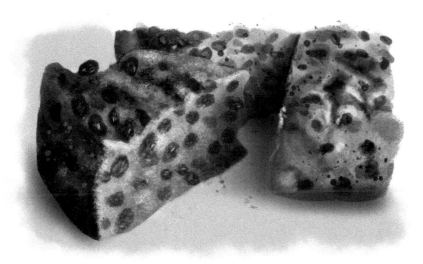

water. Pick & dry them extremely well. Take 2 pound of Double refined Sugar beet & sieved, one oz of mace shred, Half a pound of Citron cut in long thin pieces, ¼ pound of Candid Orange & as much Lemon cut in small peeces. When you begin to mix your Cake you must have a large wooden Bole ready, let it be very clean. You must poor Scalding water in to it & let it be dry & you must wash your Hands in hot water. Then take 4 pound of the Best Butter, wash it well & Beat in the bole again to get the water from it. Then Beat it 'till it looks like Cream. Strew the Sugar in by degrees & have ready 32 new laid Eggs. Beat the yolks & whites separately, the whites to a high froth & the yolks beaten but a little w'th a Gill of Sack. Put them to the butter & Sugar & beat them very well together. Put the mace in to the flour & put them in by degrees & beat it 'till it looks white, then add the whites of the Eggs.

Savoy Biscuits

Ingredients:

1lb of eggs (leaving out two yolks)
1¼lb of caster sugar, plus extra for sprinkling
Orange flower water or rosewater
¾lb of flour

Baking paper

Method: Take a pounde of Eggs & leave out the youlks of two of them then beat your Eggse very well. Then take a pound and quarter of lofe suger beten & Sieved & put into your eggs and beet it for 2 owers. Then put in a lettell Orrange flower water or rose water, whiche you like best, and three quarters of a pound of flour well dryed & beet it agane for halfe an ower. So drop them upon paper. Take care in the baken of them & sarse [sieve?] some suger on them.

A Seed Cake

Ingredients:

1 pint of cream
½ pint of ale yeast
2 eggs, separated
2 spoonsful of rose water
1¾lb of butter
3lb of flour
1 spoonful of bruised coriander seed
1 candied orange peel
2 candied citron peels
1½lb of caraway comfits

Method: Take a pint of cream, warme it & put to it half a pint of ale yeast then beate & add 2 whites, 2 yolks of eggs in 2 spoonfulls of rose water & then the cream, then melt a pound & 3 quarter of butter. Do not stir it but skim it & poure off the clear into your cream and remember to straine your butter, eggs & yeast. Have ready 3 pound of flower, a spoonful of coriander seed bruised, 1 candy orange peel, 2 of citrons peeled & mix in the flour, then put the cream to the flour & work it & set it ariseing by the fire 'till the cream be hott then work in a pound & a half of caraway comfits leaveing a few to throw on the topp. Then poure it into your coffin & bake it 3 quarters of an houre.

Seed Cake, Another

Ingredients:

2lb of flour
2lb of powdered sugar
2lb of butter
10 eggs
10 egg whites
4 ounces of caraway seeds

Method: Take 2 pound of flour and drye it in the oven and 2 pounds of powder suger and drye it well & sifte them both that there be no lumps in it. Take 2 pounds of Butter and beete it with your hands 'till it comse to Cream; 20 Eggs, halfe the whites and beete them well together for 2 owers. Strane them through a sive. Mix it well. Add 4 ounces Carraway seeds. Mix it all together then beete it then put it into your pan or cake hoop. Let it stand 2 owers in the oven.

Shortcakes

Ingredients:

3lb of butter
8 egg whites
¼lb of sugar
½lb of currants
Enough flour to make a light paste

Method: Take 3 pound of Butter & set it before the fire in a bole 'till it melts as it stands. Then beate 8 whites of Eggs & put the froth stirring upon the butter as you beate the Eggs then put in a quarter of a pound of beaten sugar & halfe a pound of Currance well Washed & dry'd in a cloth. Then mingle all this up with flour so that the past be very Light & so make Cakes of it.

Spanish Biscuits

Ingredients:

1lb of sugar, plus extra
6 eggs
4 yolks
Flour, enough to make a batter
Wine, enough to fill 2 egg shells
2 wafers

Tins, for baking

Method: Take a pound of Sugar, 10 Eggs, 4 w'th [without] the whites, the sugar beat finely & put into the eggs by litle & litle beating it together as you put it in & after it is in very strongly then take very fine flour and strew it in by little & litle continually beating it together as you put it in. After it is in very strongly then take very fine flour & strew it in by little & little – let it be but a little thicker that you make batter for pann cakes & in the beating put in as much wine as will fill two Egg shells. Then take two Wafer cakes & lay them in tin coffins & poure batter upon them then take sugar grosly beaten and strew slieght over them and when thay are halfe baked cut them into what form you please and set them into the oven again.

Wafers

Ingredients:

1lb of fine flour
¼lb of sugar
2 yolks
Milk, as much as will make a batter (the consistency of pancake
   batter)
Spices, to taste (optional)
Lemon peel (optional)

Wafer tongs

Method: Take one pounde of the Finest Flour and a quar'r of a pou'd of Lofe Sug'r beaten very fine and sersed [sieved], the yolks of two eggs well beaton and as much new milck as will mix them as stif as for a Pancake and so bake them. If you would have them taste of Spices you must boyle them in the Milck and let it be coulked agane before you mix it. If you would have it taste of Lemon, lay the peal in the milke an Houer or two before you mix them.

Wiggs

Ingredients:

2lb of flour
¼lb of butter
¼lb of sugar
Milk
Yeast
Salt

Method: Take one pound and a half of flour, one quarter of Butter and one quarter of Sugar. Moisten your Butter in Milk and put as much yeast as will make it rise then work altogether and lay it before the fire 'till it rise. Then worke half a pound of flour more in it and then role it out and lay it in a stove to rise and when they are risen put them into the oven. You must make your dough as salty as a pudding.

Cheeses, Custards and Creams

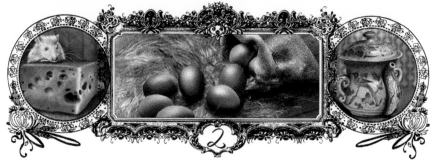

The creams prepared at Nostell had a variety of strong flavours, from the first recipe included in this selection, which was made with almonds and rose water, to *Scottish Cream*, made with nutmeg and lemon peel.

As already noted, the receipt for *Pretty Cream* includes drops of ambergris, a substance obtained from the intestines of sperm whales (but also found floating in tropical seas). In this period it was used to flavour a variety of dishes, but today survives as an ingredient used in perfumes.

The recipe for *Ramekins* requires a pound of Cheshire Cheese and a like quantity of Warwickshire Cheese. Though lesser-known these days, the latter was popular in this era, and in 1806 the novelist Jane Austen and her mother visited their relative's seat at Stoneleigh Abbey in Warwickshire, where the older lady noted in a letter that the abbey possessed a 'delightful dairy, where is made butter, good Warwickshire cheese and cream'.

The cheeses contained in Sabine's receipt books would likewise have been made on the Nostell estate, and Lady Harbord's receipt for *Marigold Cheese* required access to both a cheese cloth and a cheese press.

Sabine obviously had a well-stocked library of historical and contemporary cookbooks to refer to; indeed, one receipt, entitled *Mrs Eall's Custard*, was from a publication dating to 1718 called *Mrs Eales' Receipts* and required ten eggs, mace and a red-hot poker!

Almond Cream

Ingredients:

½lb of almonds
2 pints of cream
Rose water (to taste)
Sugar (to taste)

Method: Take half a pound of almonds & a quart of cream. Blanche your almonds & beat them very well in rose water, then strain them through a stronge strainer withe the cream (it being first boyled 'till all the rawness be out of it), then seasone it to your taste withe rose water & suger: and boyle it again 'till it thickense, then put it into your dishe to cool before you serve it up.

Apricot Custard

Ingredients:

30 apricots
1 pint of cream
8 yolks
2 egg whites
¼lb pound of sugar
2 spoonsful of rose water

Method: Take 30 Aprycoocks, pare them & stone them, cut them the longe way, & put them into the bottom of the dishe. You must have ready a quart of creame & the yolks of 8 eggs and 2 whites & beat them well with a quarter of a pound of suger & 2 spoonfulls of rose water. Stir it well with the creame, por it jeantly to your Aprycocks & bake it in a very soft oven.

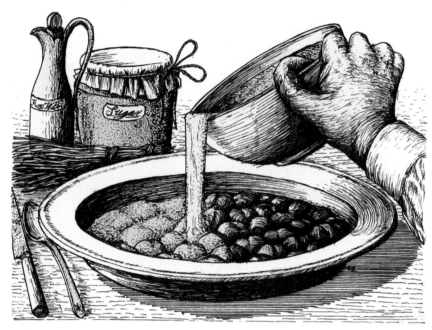

11. Apricot Custard by Peter Brears. Here peeled and stoned apricot halves are being covered with a rose water-flavoured egg custard first before being baked in a cool oven.

Barley Cream

Ingredients:

Pearl barley
Sweet cream
Isinglass
Sliced oranges or lemons

Method: Take some pearle barly, washe it in a littell fair water, then take as much sweat cream as you have yoose for. Put your barly into it and set it on the fire & let it boyle 'till it be prety thick, then put in a pease of ising glass and when it is boyled a nofe [enough] pore it into your dishe & let it stand to creame. If you like it, stick into it some sliced oranges or cittrons.

Custard

Ingredients:

2 pints of cream
4 eggs
8 yolks
Sugar, to taste
1 nutmeg

Method: To a quart of cream put 12 eggs, leave out 8 of the whites. Beat your eggs very well, then mix the eggs & cream together. Sweet'en it to your taste, then slice in a nutmeg, & then bake or boyle as you please.

Egg Cheese

Ingredients:

2 pints of new milk
3 eggs
Juice and peel of ½ a lemon
Sugar, to taste
Custard
White wine

Method: Take a Quart of new milk, take 3 Eggs, beat them very well & put them to your milk when warm & keep it stiring all the while 'till it cums to a Curd. Put in the Juice of half a lemon, a Little Sugar, put it in a collinder to drain. When the whey is all run from it, turn it out in to your Dish. Make a Custard and pour over it. Sweeten your Custard & put a piece of Lemon peal & some white wine in to it.

To make Fresh Cheese

Ingredients:

6 eggs
2 pints of cream
Rosewater, to taste
Sugar, to taste

Method: Take 6 Eggs beatte them & put them into a quart of Cream then set it on the fier keeping stiring till it begins to cruddle then tye it up in a Cloath & lett it stand 'till it be cold. Bruse it with a spoon & season it w'th Rosewater & sugar & put it into a dish & lett it stand as long as you please.

Lady Harbord's Marigold Cheese

Ingredients:

10 pints of new milk
2 pints of cream
2 good handfuls of marigold flowers
Rennet, as much as needed
Salt

Cheese cloth
Cheese press

Method: Take 5 quarts of new milke and one quarte of Cream. Then take 2 good handfulls of merygold flowers. Stamp them and strane them into the milk. Then pute in as muche rennett as you thinke fit. The milk being warmed when it is come, take up the curde and put it into a clothe to whey very tender, then put it into your Cheese vat and put a bord upon it and 3 pound waight and the next morning put it into the Chees press for one hower and when you take it out rub a littall salt on it. And so let it dry. These Cheeses will hardly be Eatabell under 6 or 8 weeks time. You must not make them 'till the Latter end of August or September.

Mrs Drake's Sack Posset

Ingredients:

10 eggs
½ a pint of sack, otherwise sherry
½lb of icing sugar
2 pints of cream

Charcoal fire

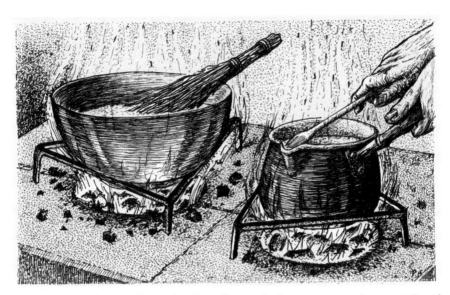

12. Mrs Drake's Sack Posset by Peter Brears. Sack posset was a hot semi-liquid smooth, rich alcoholic egg custard, the most soporific of all nightcaps. It was made by scalding the warm sherry, sugar and eggs in the silver basin with boiling cream from the saucepan.

Method: Take 10 Eggs, whites & all, & beate them in a sasepan. Then put half a pynte of sac & halfe a pounde of lofe suger, beaten [with the eggs from the saucepan], into a silver bason over a cleare charcoal fier stirin it well one waye for feare it should Curdell. Then put a quarte of cream in another sarspane over a clear fyer & let it boyle. Then when thease are just boyled take the creame off then poure it upon your Eggs into your bason then take it off frome the fire. Cover it close with a dishe & so set it upon the colde grounde & let it stande halfe an hower or more then sarve it up. Your creame & eggs must warme at one time: the creame in a sarspane & the eggs sacke & suger in a sealed bason and the bottom must be put into a stove over a carkecole fier.

Mrs Eall's Custard

Ingredients:

2 pints of cream
10 yolks
Sugar, to taste
2 blades of mace
Orange flower or rose water, to taste

Red-hot poker

Method: Take a quart of Cream, the yolks of 10 Eggs & mangel it together & sweeten it to your tast. Put in too blades of mace, a littell Orange flower or Roose water then put it on a gentill fier, sturing it till it boyls, then put them in your Cups & with a red hot shovell holde over every Cup 'till you make them look brown.

Mrs Spencer's Lemon Cream

Ingredients:

1 pint of cream, plus an extra spoonful
1 Lemon
3 egg whites
Sugar, equal to the quantity of lemon flesh, plus extra for sweetening

Method: Take a pint & a halfe of cream & set it over the fire and put into it a peece of Lemon peal cut very thin then beat the whites of 3 Eggs very well with a Spoonfull of cream and when the cream hath boyld take it off the fire and sweeteen it to your tast with Loofe sugar and put in the eggs and give it a warme on the fire. Then have a Lemon cutt very thin in round slices cut in foure peeces and strewed over with sugar so that you must put as much sugar as Lemons. Then stir it very well and set it on the fire again & let it stand for a quarter of an houre & stir it now & then but it must not be on too hot a fire for fear to make it burn. Then take it off and stirr 'till it be almost cold and then put it in your dish.

Orange Cream

Ingredients:

Juice of 6 large oranges
10 eggs
Caster or icing sugar, to taste
Butter, to taste
Cream, to taste
3 or 4 spoonsful of orange flower or rose water (optional)

Method: To 6 large Orranges add the youlk of 10 Eggs well beten. Mix your Eggs with the juse of your Orranges. Sweten it well with fine suger & then let it come through a sive. Set it over a Chafing dish, sturring it continually untill it be thick. Then put in a littell pease of butter & when it is melted take it off the fire & store it 'till it is cold. Then have redy some cold cream (having previously been boiled). Sweten it with fine suger and mix together to your taste. If you like the taste you may put in 3 or 4 spoone fulls of Orrange flower or roos water.

Pretty Cream

Ingredients:

1 pint of cream
7 egg whites
Sugar, to taste
2 or 3 bay leaves
5 or 6 drops of ambergris
Tarts, to serve

Method: Take a pint of Cream, 7 whites of Eggs, Sugar to your Tast, 2 or 3 Bay-leafes. Set your Cream on the Fire 'till 'tis warm, then put in the rest of your Things, stirring it till it is thick. Just before you take it off put in 5 or 6 drops of amb'r grease then put it into high sweetmeat Glasses & when cold set it amongst Tarts or by Themselves.

Ramekins

Ingredients:

1lb of Cheshire cheese
1lb of Warwickshire cheese
1 or 2 spoonsful of cream
French bread
Butter, for greasing
Burning charcoal

Method: Take a pound of good old Cheese Cheshire and a pound of good Warwickshire Cheese, only the inside, and beat them together in a Morter with a spoonfull or two of Cream. Toast some French bread and put your Cheese thereon pretty thick & having Buttered the bottom of a dish set your Ramkins in it then take a potting pan covered with some Charcoal on the top to brown them and so serve them up as hot as you can.

Scottish Cream

Ingredients:

Thick cream
1 nutmeg
Lemon juice, as much as will curdle the cream
Sugar, to taste

Method: Take thick cream and boyle it with as much more. Take a nutmeg quartered, it will give it a pretty taste, then take it of and let it stand 'till it be warm then straine it into as much juice of Lemon, or for want of that as much will Crudle [curdle] it then sweeten it with sugar and let it stand 'till it be cold and serve it up unbroken.

Tea Cream

Ingredients:

2 pints of cream
Sugar, to taste
¼oz of tea
Inward skins of chickens

Tea cup
Hot cinders

Method: Take a Quart of Cream, set it over the Fire, sweeten to your
tast, add a Quarter of an Oz of Tea. Let your Tea Boyl in your Cream
& keepe it stirring 'till it has taken the tast of the Tea. Then take it off
the Fire. Then take the inward skin of Chickens, wash them Clean, Cut
them Small, put them in a Tea Cup & fill it up w'th the Tea Cream. Set
the Cup near the 'fire till it comes then put it to your Cream & strain it
off two or three times. Set the dish you will serve it up in near the Fire
& if you have a tin cover lay some hot sinders on the Top. After it is a
little come set it to Coal & serve it up. Coffee Cream is made the same
way.

Jams, Jellies, Pickles and Preserves

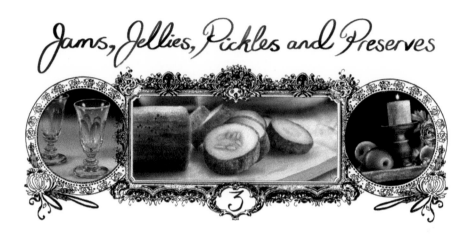

Preserving and pickling was certainly popular in this period and the receipt books are full of such entries, with quaint titles like *The Very Old Way of Preserving Cherries* or *Preserve Goosberries as Green as they Grow*. But of course, with abundant gardens and orchards, and the expense of obtaining ingredients from distant markets and dealers, preservation was an essential part of the overall management of the household kitchen, especially given the limited seasonal availability of certain fruits and other food. And the use of salt and sugar meant that food lasted longer and strong flavours were retained.

Although only a selection of these is included, the receipt books illustrate that quite a wide variety of food was being consumed. Included here are instructions on how to pickle Indian pepper, button mushrooms and cucumbers, whilst the range of preserves stretches to apples, plums, oranges, peascods and peaches, the latter which could be made into a syrup if Sir Theodore Colladon's recipe was followed.

And as well as receipts for *Raspberry Jelly* and *White Quince Marmalade*, this selection even includes a recipe for *Walnut Ketchup*. But it is perhaps most noteworthy for the receipt for *Pickled Cabbage*. This is actually a recipe for the Swiss/German dish *sauerkraut*, which was not common in eighteenth-century England. It was perhaps a favourite of Sabine's from her time in her home country of Switzerland.

Green Apple Preserve

Ingredients:

Pippins
1lb 2oz of sugar for every lb of apples
1 pint of water for every 1lb 2oz of sugar
1 egg white

Method: In July take pipins & put them into a basin or Skillett full of Water & cover them close. Let the dish keep them under water. Set them on a Temperate fier that the water may be never hotter than you enduer to touch it. Remove the pippins and peel them, and then put them in the water again, & as you peel them keep them close covered 'till they be as green as grass. Then take them & weigh them, & to every pound of Apples take a pound & 2 ounces of Sugar then put them in the same water again & then let them lye 'till you have made your sirup. To a pound & 2 ounces of Sugar you must take a pint of water. Clarify your sirup with the white of an Egg & boyle your sirup. Then cut your apples to the core on one side & so boile them in the sirup. Lett your sirup be cold & your green fruit must not boile so long in the sirup for that will make them look a Russet colour. The beginning of August is the best time to do the pipins.

Green Plum Preserve

Ingredients:

Largest green and hard plums
2lb of double refined sugar for every 2lb of plums
½ a pint of water for every 2lb of plums
½lb of codling apple jelly
½lb of sugar

Method: Take the Largest plums when green & hard & set a thing of water over the fire. When it boils take it off & let it stand a very little while, then put in your plums, cover them close & lett them stand halfe a quarter of an houre. Then take them out off that water & put them in such another water & cover them close, letting them stand a Little while then see if the skinn will peel. If the skin do not rise put them in another water & let them stand a While Close covered, then peel them & as you do soe put them in a thing of hott water and when all are peel'd cover them close & lett them stand on a Little fire but have a care they do not boile & so lett them stand 'till they are green then take them out of the water & to two pounds of plums take 2 pounds of Sugar double Refin'd finely beaten & a pint & a halfe of water. Put the sugar & water together in a Basin of silver. Leave a Little of the Sugar out to strew on as they boile. Set them on a quick fire & make them boile with all speed. When you see them look clear & that they are almost done put in halfe a pound of Jelly of Codling and half a pound of Sugar & then let it boile 'till you see it as a Jelly. Then take them up in Glasses & keep them all the year.

India Pickles [Piccalilli]

Ingredients:

½lb of ginger
Salt
Water
½lb of garlic
1oz of long pepper
1oz of bruised mustard seeds
½oz of turmeric
1 gallon of good vinegar
Pickles in the form of raw cauliflower florets, white cabbage, small cucumbers, radishes, kidney beans, beetroot etc.

Method: Take half a pound of Ginger, let it lie in Salt & Water one night, then scrape it & cut it in thin slices. Put it in a Jar with dry Salt & let it stand till the rest of your Ingredients are ready. Take half a pound of Garlick, peel it, slice it & salt it for 3 days then wash it & salt it 3 days more. Wash it again & put it in a Sieve to dry in the Sun. Take one ounce of long Pepper, wash it & salt it, put it in the Sun to dry, but not too much. One Ounce of mustard seed bruised very fine & half an Ounce of Turmerick. Put all these together in a stone Jar, boil a gallon of good Vinegar & put to it. When cold brine your Pickles with a strong Brine, boiling hot. You may put in every thing but Walnuts & need ever empty your Jar.

Mrs Fortescue's Gooseberries

Ingredients:

Gooseberries
Sugar

Preserving glasses

Method: Take the fairest & largest gooseberryes and stoan them & then put them into a glass of faire water then take other gooseberryes & when they are stewed pour the Liquor from them into preserveing glasses. Then put more gooseberryes into the cann & do with them as with the former until you have syrup enough for the ston'd gooseberries. Then to two pound of sirup you may put one pound of sugar & to one pound of stewed Gooseberryes you may put one pound of Sugar & one pound of stewed gooseberrys. You must put three quarters of a pound of Sugar but you must boyle it up to a candy then take your gooseberrys out of the water & put them into the sugar as it boiles on the fier and strew & scum them. They must boile as fast as thay can & when thay are allmost ready put to the sirup of Gooseberyes with the rest of the sugar into the basen on the fier & so let them boile together and skimme them very well and then put them into glasses & sprinkle with sugar. It must be very fine sugar.

Mrs Winn's Pickled Mushrooms

Ingredients:

Mushrooms
Milk
Salt
Vinegar
White wine
White pepper
2 or 3 cloves
Ginger, to taste
Olive oil

Method: Take mushoromse of a nice grothe, cut off the stalks then put them in water then wipe them clean and change your water 3 or 4 timse. Boyle them in milke and water and a littell salte. Skim them very cleane. A quarter of an ower will boyle them. Put them into a sieve to drane. When thay are cold washe them in a littell vinegar and of white wine of eache an equell quantity. The wine & vineger you put to them must not be boyled as other pickells, just to be hot. Put to them raw. Add a littell white pepper, 2 or 3 cloves & jeanger to your tast. When the bottell is full put on oyell on the top. Cover it close for your use.

Orange and Lemon Marmalade

Ingredients:

Oranges
Fine sugar (double the weight of the fruit peels)
Pippin pulp

Method: Take the best fair-skin'd Oranges & cut 'em into halves. Squeeze out the Juice into a little Bason & rub the peals with salt in a course cloth, & boyle 'em in 3 waters as you do whole oranges, & when they are tender, take out the pulp & weigh the peals. Take double their weight in fine sugar, & make a little pulp of Pippins to melt then shred your Orange-peals or slice 'em very thin & put 'em to your sugar, & let 'em boyle well together 'till they are pretty stiff. And so pour it into Glasses or Pots for Marmalade. You may put some of the juice into the Marmalade as it is boyleing with as much Sugar as you think fit.

Pickled Artichokes

Ingredients:

Globe artichokes
Pickling liquor (made to your preferred recipe)

Leather, for covering

Method: Take the Heartychookes and cut the Leaves off round but not too close. Then boil them about a quarter of an hour and then try one or two in some cold water to see whether the Choke will rub off then put them in Cold watter and shift them two or three times in fresh watter that day, then make your Pickle [of salt and water] as strong as will bear an Egg, & boil it & let it stand to be Quiet [quite?] Cold before you put it to your Heartychokes. You may let the Choks be on if you please. Cover them with a Leather. Sometimes they will be ropy in a Month or 2. If so you must wash them Clean & boil the same pickle up again & let it stand to be cold.

Pickled Button Mushrooms

Ingredients:

Button mushrooms
Spring water
Dry salt
White wine vinegar
White wine
Large mace
Allspice
Ginger

Method: Gather the little white Buttons & as soon as you bring 'em in put 'em into a great deal of Spring water then take dry salt & rub every one severall on the top with your Thumb 'till they are very white & as you do 'em fling 'em one by one into another vessel full of Spring water. When your Quantity is done you must take 'em out & boyle 'em for half an hour in another water puting into it a good quantity of salt then set 'em to drain on the top of a Sieve & when they are cold have a pickle ready to put 'em in made of white wine vinegar & white wine according as you would have it for sharpness in w'ch you must boyle some large mace, Jamaca pepper & a few bits of Ginger. The Pickle must be cold & before you put in the Mushrooms keep 'em close stopped in a wide mouth'd Glass. You may boyle the Mushrooms at severall times as you can gather 'em but be sure you let 'em be cold before you put 'em into the Pickle, that the other is in. The quicker they are done after they are gathered the better.

Pickled Cabbage [Sauerkraut]

Ingredients:

Salt
Juniper berries
Caraway seeds
Cabbage, including the leaves

1 large tub, well pitched
1 board as large as the mouth of the tub
1 heavy weight
Clean linen cloths

Method: You must have a tub well pitched in the bottom. Lay a handfull of salt, some juniper berries and caraway seeds then lay on a good quantity of Cabbage cut in slices. Press it down hard with your hands 'till it yealds. Then lay salt, Juniperberres and caraway seeds as before & then cabage and still pressing it down, this done 'till the tub

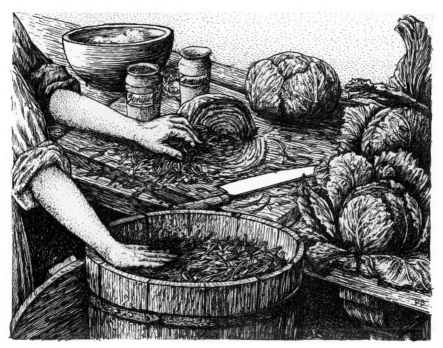

13. Sauerkraut by Peter Brears. Sauerkraut, a form of fermented shredded cabbage, was introduced to Nostell by Sabine Winn from her native Switzerland.

be full, then lay on it cabage Leaves and a board as big as the top of the mouth of the tubb and a great weight. Thus let it stand 9 or 10 days to work. When it hath done working take off the cabage leaves & instead of them lay on a clean linnen cloth and put on the board & weight and let it stand a month & then it will be fit to eat.

Pickled Cucumbers

Ingredients:

Large cucumbers
Onions
Salt
White wine vinegar
Allspice, to taste
Cloves, to taste
Mace, to taste
Whole white peppercorns, to taste

Method: Take your cucumbers and slice them into thick slices and slice a good many onyons among them, then salt them very well and set them to draine the water from them foure dayes. Then make a pickle for them of good white wine vinegar and Jamaca paper [i.e. allspice] and cloves and mace and whole white pepper and salt. It must be as strong a pickle as for small cucumbers. Then put your cucumbers and onyons alltogether into a deep pot and poure your pickle boyling hot upon them, and stop them close for 4 days. Then boyle your pickle againe and poure on them and stop them close and in a weeks time you may eate of them if you please but the longer they are kept the better.

Pickled Indian Pepper

Ingredients:

Indian peppers [red or green capsicums]
Raw vinegar

Method: Gather the peppers when at the full growth, and put them into raw vinegar, wipeing them with a clean cloth. Cover them close and let them stand 15 days then pouer off the pickle into a clean bras skillet and boile it. Let it stand 'till cold and so 'till Green. The Red is done the same way only Boill the pickle in a Silver thing if you have it. 3 or 4 times is enough for it to be boil'd for the Red.

Pippin Marmalade

Ingredients:

1¼lb of sugar
1 pint of water
1 pound of pippins
10 lemons (the juice of two and the peels of all ten)
10 oranges (the juice of one and the peels of all ten)

Method: Take one pounde of the best Suger & one pint of water and make a syrup of it, then waye one pound of pipenns & cut them in quarter & cut out the core then boyle the syrup and skim it. Then put in the pippens & let them boyle as fast as thay can. Whenn you see the pippens look clean then put in the juse of 2 lemonse & one orrange thickened with one quarter of a pound of lofe suger. Then have ready the peelles of ten lemons & orranges boyled in severall waters & cut into small bitts, and put them in a littell before you take them off. You may try a lettell in a spone & see if it comes clean from the bottom of the skillet.

To Preserve Gooseberries as Green as they Grow

Ingredients:

Green gooseberries
Water
Pre-made syrup
1 egg white

Method: Take of the fairest green gooseberries you can get and put them into hott watter and let them stand a little. Then put them away and put them into hott scalding watter and let them stand as mutch longer as before. Then take them oute and cut off the tops and peel the thin skin of them and let them stand and scald on the fire a good while. Then let them boyle a little while & then make your syrup and Clarrefie it with the white of an Egg and take your Gooses oute of the watter and put them into the syrup and let them boyle softly 'till they be very tender and Greene and so put them into your pot and boyle the syrup till it will Gelley a little. Then so put it into your Goosberrys and keep them.

A Way to preserve Green Pippins

Ingredients:

Kentish pippins
Water
Green wheat
1¼lb of double refined sugar for every pound of pippins
Gooseberry jelly or white currant jelly

Method: Take of the Right Kentish pipins and coddle them in Scolding water haveing 2 skillits on the fire at a time & when they are scalded enough peele them and cut out the black coars [cores] and put them into the fresh scalding water & let them be covered close with a plate so that all the aples be covered with water. They must be shifted 'till they be fully green, 4 or 5 times will be enough. If your aples be tender & apt to break put in a little green wheat into the water they were first scalded in & so green them. To one pound of these pipins take one & a quarter of Duble Refind sugar and make a Sirup & put the aples in & boyle them very fast and when thay are halfe done take them off & skin them well and cover them up and boyle them again the next day. All aples are apt to thin their sirup therefore you must put either Jelly of Gooseberries or white currance into them and so warm them alltogether & then put them into your glass.

Preserve Oranges

Ingredients:

1lb of prepared oranges
1½lb of sugar, plus extra
Salt
Spring water
Pippin jelly

Clean coarse cloth
Jam jars

Method: Take the greate high coloured orinyes. Pare them very thin and rub them with salt and lay them in spring water 2 or 3 days, shifting them 2 or 3 times a day. Then boyle them in 3 waters 'till they are very tender. Before you boyle them make a hole in the top of the orange and take out all the seeds. When they are boyled very tender lay them on a clean cours cloath with the holes downe & let all the water runn clear from them. Then make a sirup of them: thus to a pound of orinyes take a pound & a halfe of Sugar & half a pint of water. Let your Sorup boyle then put in your orinyes & let them boyle as fast as possible. As they boyle strew in now and then some sugar which you must keep out when you make the sirup. When you see them cook very clear and that thay are very tender then take them up and put them in Glasses without any of the Sirup which they are boyl'd in. Take all that, as clean from the orinyes as possible you can, then fill up your Glasses with pippin Jelley.

Preserve Peascods

Ingredients:

Peascods
Sugar (the same weight as the prepared peascods), plus extra
Spring water
Rose water
Orange juice
1 cinnamon stick
Cloves

Method: Gather your peascodds whilst they be green, young & tender. Pick them & put them into a pipken of hot water & set it on the Embers covered, & so let them stand 'till they will pill [peal]. The greenest pease will do best when pilled [pealed]. Boyle them in the water they were scalded in but let it boyle before you put them in & when they look green and tender take them up. And when they be cold weigh them and take their weight in sugar and put a Little spring water to it and let it boyle. Scum it cleane and put a Little rosewater to it & let it boyle to a Surup. Then take it off & when it is all most cold put in your peascodds & let them boyle whilst they be tender. Then take them up but let the Sirup boyle longer. When it is cold put to the peascodds

& so let it stand six or seven dayes cloase covered then poure out the sirup into a silver dish adding thereto according to your quantity the Juice of orinrges & a Little fine sugar, a stick of sinimon & a few cloves & so boyle it to pretty thick sirup scumming it very clean thirce. When it is cold put in your peascodds.

Ripe Plums

Ingredients:

1lb of plums
1lb of sugar

Preserving pan
Jam jars, or similar

Method: To 1 p'd of Plumbs put 1 p'd of Sug'r. Wett the sug'r in watt'r & just boil itt up & skim itt & slitt the plumbs on the sides & put 'em into a Pott till the next day. Poor the liq'r from them & heat it scalding hott & put to them againe & cover them. This do 2 or 3 times to keep the skin on them. Put them in a broad preserveing pan & boil them 'till they will Jelly, then glass them.

Sir Theodore Colladon's Peach Flower Syrup

Ingredients:

3lb of peach flowers or blossoms
2 pints of boiling water
1½lb of double refined sugar (to each pound of liquor)

Method: Take peach flowers or blossoms one pound, pour over them a Quart of boyleing hott wotter. Let it stand aboute 12 hours then straine it then warme it againe boyleing hott and pour it over as many flowers as before. Thus do three times and to each pound of the liquor put a pound and half of double refin'd sugar and boyle it up in to the consistance of syrup, that is about a Quarter of an houre upon a Gentle fire.

The 'Very Old' Recipe for Raspberry Jelly

Ingredients:

Fresh raspberries

White currants

1lb of beaten sugar for every pint of liquor obtained from the
currants

Jam jars, or similar

Method: Take Rasberres freashe gather'd & white corranse. Strim the
curranse and bruise them together & put them over the fier & boyl
them a pretty whille. Then strane them throw a fine straner. Then for
every pint of liquor add one pound of beaten suger & so boyle it 'till it
comes to a jealy & so glase it for your youse.

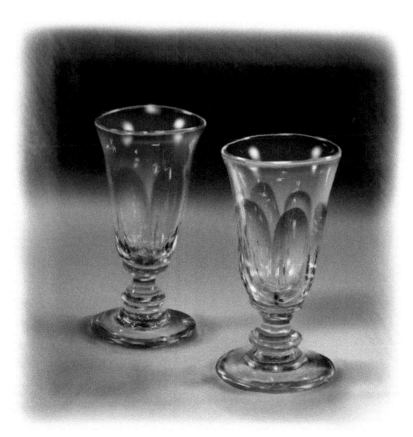

The 'Very Old' Way of Preserving Cherries

Ingredients:

1lb of stoned cherries
1lb of sugar
12 spoonsful of currant juice

Jam jars

Method: To one pound of Cherres Stoned, one pound of Suger and 12 spone fulls of the juse of Curanse. Put thease in a pan and at first let it boyle lesuerly then make it boyle as fast as you can & skim it some timse & when you think it will jealy & the Cherres look Cleen, take them off the fier & pot them in pots or glasses.

Walnut Ketchup

Ingredients:

Fresh walnuts, enough to obtain 2 pints of juice
1 pint of alegar, otherwise beer vinegar
1 handful of salt
Cloves, to taste
Mace, to taste
Nutmeg, to taste
Black pepper, to taste

Stone bottle

Method: Gather your walnuts when they are fit for pickling. Pound them in a stone mortour. Strain out the Juice and to every Quart put a Pint of Alegar & a hand full of Salt. Let it stand 24 hours then Pour it off clear. Simmer it over a Slow fire 'till half is Wasted then put it into a Stone Bottle and to it Cloves, Mace & Nutmeg Sliced and add black Pepper according to your judgment.

White Quince Marmalade

Ingredients:

1lb of peeled and cored quinces
1lb of sugar
1 spoonful of water

Jars

Method: Pare & core your quinses & to every pound of quince one pound of Suger. Put your quinces & suger together & one sponefull of water & set it on the fier and let your suger be melted before you let it boyle. Then let it boyle as fast as you can 'till it comes from the botome of your pane & so put it in your pots.

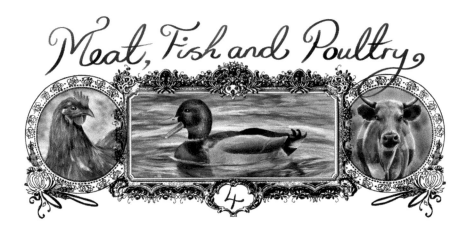

Meat, Fish and Poultry

4

Whilst Sabine's receipt books contain several recipes for beef dishes, there is also quite a variety of different meats, fish and poultry to try. These include mutton, hare, turkey, oysters, bacon and even Westphalian ham, these being pigs reared on acorns in the Westphalian forests of north-western Germany. Several ingredients could be obtained locally, from Nostell's own estates in some cases, but obviously if Westphalia ham was ever on the menu, it suggests a wider network of procurement.

An advert in the *Manchester Mercury* newspaper on 30 March 1790 offered Westphalia Ham for sale at Burgess's Warehouse at 107 Corner of the Savoy Steps, Strand, London: 'To the CURIOUS in HAMS, TONGUES, &c. A large Quantity of exceedingly fine flavoured WESTMORELAND and WESTHPHALIA HAMS, such as may be depended on to please every taste.' This establishment, founded by John Burgess at 101 the Strand in 1774, would perhaps have been familar to the Winns, who had a property at St James's Square in Westminster at this time, which was less than a mile away.

Burgess, who became famous for producing an anchovy sauce, stated in his advertisement that he received 'generous patrongage', from members of the 'nobility, gentry and others'.

As with the previous selection, preservation was important and there are two recipes for potted dishes: hare and lobster whereby the hare or lobster would be packed into a pot, typically made of earthenware, and sealed inside with butter or fat. In the case of the lobster recipe, a large weight was required to ensure it was well packed in the pot. Potting would allow food that would otherwise quickly perish to be kept for many weeks.

Bake a Leg of Mutton

Ingredients:

Leg of mutton
2 yolks
2 or 3 spoonsful of white wine vinegar
¼ pint of red wine
Salt and pepper, to taste

Method: Cut out the bone & beet your meet very well, then take the youlke of 2 Eggs with 2 or 3 spoonefulls of white wine Vinegar & mingell it with halfe a pint of Red wine & pour it to your meet & rub it well inn. Seson it withe pepper & salt & the next day turne, & the morning after bake it.

Buttered Chicken

Ingredients:

1 whole chicken
1 cold, roasted whole chicken
2 pints of water
1 blade of mace
Salt and pepper, to taste
Grated bread
¼ pint of fresh butter
1 lemon

Method: Take a chicken and cut it into peeses and boyle it in a quart of water with a blade of mase & a littel salt 'till it 'tis very good broth. Then take a Cold Chicking that has bin Rosted and take all the skin off and cut it into pieces and put some of your Broth into it and Season it with peper and salt and put some grated Bread into it to thicken it. When it is stewed anuf put a quartern [quarter of a pint] of fresh butter into it and squese a whole lemon into it and season it to your Taste.

Creamy Chicken Pie

Ingredients:

1 chicken
Pastry
Mushrooms
Oysters
Morels
Salt and pepper, to taste
Cullis à la Reine
Juice of 1 lemon

Method: Cut your Chicken in four. Lay them in to your Pastry w'th mushrooms, oysters & morels. Put in seasoning to your [taste]. Just when Bak'd cut off the Lid & put in a Cullis ala Reign w'th the Juice of a Lemon. White Gravy will do very well.

Galantine of Rabbits

Ingredients:

Rabbits (as many as needed)
Pepper, to taste
Salt, to taste
Sweet herbs, to taste
Thin slices of bacon (with equal amounts of fat and lean meat)
Veal and beef suet
Butter, for basting
Ragù sauce, for serving
Mushrooms or morels, for serving
Sliced lemon, for garnish

Packthread, for tying

Method: Bone the Rabits, beat them flat, season them w'th Pepper, Salt and Sweet herbs, then take some thin Slices of Bacon, mix't fat & lean, & make a forcemeat w'th Veale & Beef Suit. Spread the forcemeat over the Rabits & the Bacon upon it then role the Rabits very tite. Tye them round in 4 Places at an Equal Distance with Pack thread. Spit

& Roast them. Bast them very well w'th butter. Serve them up w'th a Ragoo Sauce. You may add moshrooms, morels or any other thing you like. Garish w'th slic'd Lemon.

How to Roast a Rump of Beef

Ingredients:

Sweet marjoram
Thyme
Winter savory
Marrow or beef suet
Rump of beef
Claret wine
Shallots

Method: Take some Sweat Margarum & time & winter Savory & shred them small with some marrow or beaf suet, & stuff the beaf with it. Then baste the beaf with clarat wine & save all that drops from it & when you serve it up pore your fatt a way and put your gravey into the dish for sase [sauce]. If you pleas you may rub the dish with sharlot.

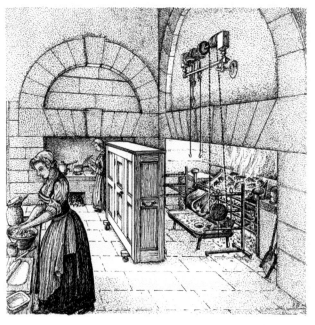

14. Roasting by Peter Brears. The smoke jack that still remains in Nostell's kitchen was powered by a large round fan mounted within the chimney flue. It turned joints of meat mounted on spits set before the radiant coal fire, the cupboard-like roasting screen being lined with shining tinplate to reflect the heat onto the meat, and protect the cooks.

Meat Patties

Ingredients:

Roasted white meat, minced
Suet, as much to make the meat moist
Thyme, to taste
Onions, to taste
Pepper, to taste
Salt, to taste
1 or 2 yolks
Puff pastry
Dripping, for frying

Method: Mince any sort of white meat very fine after it has been
Roasted & as much suet as will make it verry moist. Season it with a
little time, onions and pepper, & salt to your Taste. Add the yolk of an
Egg or two, according to your quantity, & put it into puff paste Roll'd
very thinn. Fry it in Boyling hot dripping.

Mother's Scotch Collops

Ingredients:

1 leg of veal
Anchovies
White wine
½ pint gravy
3 yolks
Butter
Bacon
Sausage balls

Method: Take a Leg of Veal & cut your Collops very thin then clop
'em with the back of a knife, then put 'em into a Frying-pan with a little
water & fry 'em 'till they are almost enough, turning 'em often, that they
may not harden. Then put in a little Anchovie & white wine & when
enough put in half a pint of Gravey, the yolks of 3 eggs, well beaten &
mingled together, & some butter. Stir 'em well in the pan that the eggs

may not curdle, then take it from the fire & shake the meat & sauce together then put it into the dish with some thin bits of fry'd Bacon & Sassage balls to lay about it.

Mrs Eall's Mumbled Hare

Ingredients:

Hare
12 eggs
Sweet herbs
1lb of butter
Seasoning, to taste

Method: Take your hare & boil it then Cut the flesh of the bons adding 12 eggs, a litel sweet herbs. Fried all theas very well to gether then put it in a sawes pan adding a pound of buter & be sure you seasen it to your tast then sarve it up.

Mrs Thornhill's Chicken Fricassee

Ingredients:

Whole chickens (as many as needed)
Lemon peel, to taste
Mace, to taste
Pepper, to taste
Cream, as needed
White wine, to taste
Lemon juice, to taste
A lump of butter
Flour
Pickled mushrooms, to garnish
Morels, to garnish

Method: Boil your Chickings almost enough then flee [flay] them & cut them into handsome Pieces. Shred some lemon Peal, a little mace & pepper and strew it on them as much as you think will season them.

Take the Bones of the Chickings & strew them in some of the Liquor they were Boyld in. Put in a Blade of mace & a piece of Lemon peal. Let it stew some time, then strainit into a Sause pan with as much Cream as will toss it up. Put in a little White Wine & a little Lemon Juice & a lump of Butter rold in Flower to make it a good thickness. You may add Pickl'd mushrooms & morels just as you serve it up.

Mutton Rumps

Ingredients:

6 or 8 mutton rumps
Butter, for frying and thickening the sauce
Slices of:
    Veal
    Beef
    Mutton
    Ham
Onion, to taste
Thyme, to taste
Parsley, to taste
Sweet basil or bay leaves, to taste
Homemade brown gravy (made from the above meat and
    ingredients)
Flour, for thickening the sauce
Lemon juice

Method: Take 6 or 8 mutton Rumps & fry 'em in butter until light brown. Have ready a Stewpan. At the bottom layeth slices of Veal, Beaf, mutton & ham. Lay the Rumps upon it & lay some on the top. Lay on some slices of Onion, Thyme, Parsley & Sweet Basill, if you can get it. If not, bay leaves [will do]. Put in water enough to cover them. Let 'em stew 8 howers jentley over a Slow fire, then take them out & put them into brown gravy made of the same meat & Ingredients as before. Let 'em stew an Hour then Thicken the Sause with Butter & Flour. Put in a Little Juice of Lemon.

Oyster Loaves

Ingredients:

3 anchovies
2 pints of middling oysters
14 whole peppercorns
6 cloves
2 large blades of mace
1 glass of sack or white wine
Winter savory, to taste
Thyme, to taste
Piece of butter, plus extra for basting
Breadcrumbs
6 French loaves
Greens, to serve

Method: Take 3 Anchovies, dissolve 'em in half a quart'r of a pint of Fair water, then put to your Liquor ab't a Quart of midling Oysters w'th 14 whole pepper-cornes, 6 cloves & 2 large blades of mace & a Glass of Sack or white wine (w'ch you please), a little winter savory & Thyme, shred very small, & so boyle 'em up w'th a good peice of Dish Butter & some Crumbs of bread. Put the herbs in when almost boyl'd enough, then take 6 French Loaves, cut a piece out of the top of 'em & take out all the Crumbs & so set 'em to the Fire to crisp, turning & baisting 'em w'th Fresh butter & when they are throughly hot & crisp fill 'em w'th the Stewed Oysters & lay the tops of the Loaves on again & serve 'em up garnishing your dish w'th Greens.

Oyster Pie

Ingredients:

24 pints of oysters
Seasoning, to taste
10 or 12 eggs
Bacon
Pastry, for the pie (made to any chosen recipe)
Gravy, for serving
Butter, for serving

Method: Take a peck & a halfe of Oysters, open them & washe them. Scalde them a littell & season them. Take 10 or 12 eggs & boyle them harde & cut the yolke in the middell in 2 peases. Then take a pease of fine bacon & slise it thin & laye it under the Oysters in the bottom of the pye then mix the Oysters with the yolks of the eggs & laye them in the pye & lay some thin slises of bacon on the tip of the pye and so bake it. Serve it up with some of its own licker & some gravy and butter.

Pickled Westphalian Ham

Ingredients:

Westphalian ham
1oz saltpeter
½oz sal prunella
2lb white salt
½lb brown sugar

Method: Take an Ounce of Salt peter & half an Ounce of sal-prunella, 2 pound of White salt & half a pound of Brown Sugar. Mix 'em together then salt it well & turn it every day. Let it lye a Fortnight then hang it up to dry. Leave out the Sugar when you do Tongues. Note: if you do not love your Ham dry'd, you may let it lye in the Pickle till you use it.

Pork Sausages

Ingredients:

3lb of lean, minced pork
2lb of fat
1lb of hog's suet
Pepper, to taste
Salt, to taste
Cloves, to taste
Mace, to taste
1 handful of sage
5 yolks
12 spoonsful of cream
Butter, for frying

Skins

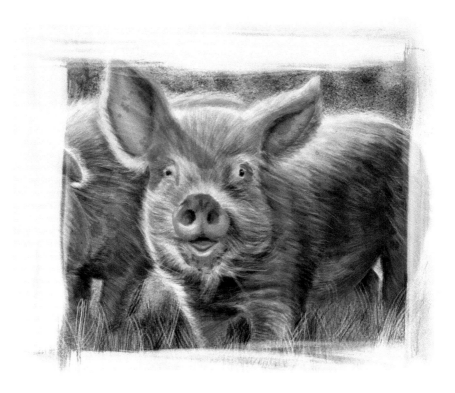

Method: Take three pound of Leane Porke. Pick it clean from the sinews and mince them very small. Then take too pound of very fine fat & one pound of hogs suet & chop them together 'till they be fine. Season them with peper and salt & cloves and mace beaten. Put in as much more cloves and mace as peper & a handful of sage shred very small, five yealks of Eggs, 12 spoonfuls of Creamm. Work it in your hand untill it be mingled. Stuff it into the skins. Frye them very Leasurely with good store of sweet Butter.

Potted Hare

Ingredients:

1 large hare, whole
Salt
Allspice, to taste
1lb of cooked bacon, including the fat
1½lb of butter

Pepper, to taste
Cloves, to taste
Nutmeg, to taste
Mace, to taste
Clarified butter

Method: Take a large Hare & cutt in pieies & put it into a Pott with a little water & salt and a little allspice & bake it all night. When you take it out of the oven lay it in a Cullender & drain it very dry. Then pick it clean from the skin & bones and shred it so fine that it will sift. Shred also a Pound of Fatt Bacon, Then beat 'em together in a stone mortar 'till it come to a Past. Then put it into a Skillet with a pound & a half of Sweet Butter. Season it with Pepper, Salt, Cloves, Nutmegg & Mace to your Tast. Keep it stirring all the while 'till it is throughly mix't. Then put it into Potts and when cold cover it with clarified Butter. This way does any sort of meat that is Roasted also.

Potted Lobster

Ingredients:

Large lobsters
Salt, to taste
Mace, to taste, or pepper, to taste
Butter
White bread

Large weight, for pressing
Pots, for potting

Method: Take the Largest Lobsters you can get. Half Boile them then take out the white part cleen from the Shels. Wipe them cleen. Season them with Salt & mace if you like that Tast. If not, with Peper. Put your Lobster in pots: a Layer of Lobster & another of Butter till your Pot is full. Put it in the Oven with White Bread & if your Pot is Large it must stay in an Hour & a half. When you take it out drain the Butter from it then Lay on a large weight to press it down then drain it again 'till all the Liquor is from it. Then take out the Lobster as whole as you can & put it in to the Pots you intend to Keepe it in but the Lobster must be put down very close in the Pots or it will not keepe. Then you must strain your Butter that your Lobster was Baked in through a Sive & put it in to the Pots.

Roast Duck

Ingredients:

Ducks
Young sage
Parsley
Winter savory
Onions
Butter
White pepper
Salt
Sliced beef
Strong broth
Thyme
1 glass of claret

Method: Put within the Ducks to Roste a little young saige, a little parcille, a little winter savery and Onyon. Shred them all a little together then take a peice of butter with white pepper beaton small & a littel salt. Mixe the herbs & butter like a peice of past and put into Every Duck the Bigness of a small Egg. For the sause take some Beef slis'd thin bryled [broiled] very brown then have ready some strong broth. Then put this in w'th an onyone, a little parcille & time. Let this Boyle well together until 'tis Strong & browne. Then strain it off then have ready Some Onyons heads boyl'd white. Cut them small mix them w'th a little thick butter then mix the Gravy w'th a glass of Clarret & let it be thick.

Stew a Calf's Head

Ingredients:

1 calf's head
2 pints of white wine
Salt, to taste
Whole pepper, to taste
2 or 3 blades of mace
3 anchovies
1 bundle of sweet herbs
1 onion, whole
Sausages
Oysters, stewed
Butter
2 yolks
Bacon
Sweetbread (optional)
Lamb testicles (optional)
Cockscombs (optional)
Puff pastry (optional)
Flour (optional)
Egg whites (optional)
Chopped sage (optional)
Spice, for seasoning (optional)
Veal balls, for serving (optional)
Nutmeg, for seasoning (optional)
Currants (optional)

Method: Take a Calfes head halfe boyl'd & then take one halfe of the head & the tongue & cut them into slices Very thin. Then put it into your stewpan with a q't of white wine & as much water as will sarve to cover the meat. Then season it with some salt, some whole peper, 2 or 3 blades of mace, 3 Anchovas, a Bundle of sweet herbs & a whole onion. Keep it close covered & let it be stewing 'till it be enough keeping the other halfe head at the fire aroasting without stewing. Cut some sausages in & have some oysters Ready stew'd & put in when tis enough. Take up your Liquor pretty thick with butter & the yolks of 2 Eggs then garnish your

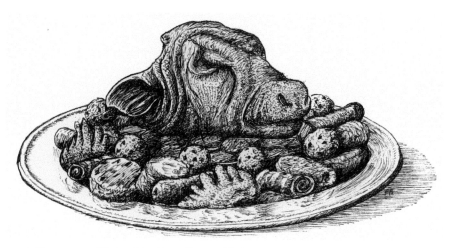

15. To stew a calf's head by Peter Brears. Today we are far more squeamish than our Georgian ancestors. This roasted calf's head was mounted on a bed of stewed slices of head and garnished with cocks' combs, bacon, sausages, oysters, veal balls and calf brains made into fried cakes and puffs.

dish w'th fry'd bacon and oysters stewed & a good many sausages with the braines made up in Little puffs & fried in butter. You may put sweet breads & Lam stoans if you can get them or Pallat [pullet] or coxcomes & you may make a great many pretty things to garnish the dish with. All the braines you may ether stew with the meat, or you may beat them with some flour & whites of eggs & chopped sage, season them with salt and spice & drop them into the pan and frye them, or if you please you may make puff past & put them in & frie them. To garnish the dish you must put the roasted half in the midle of the dish & put the stewed halfe about with sausages & oysters & the rest of the things. This is a delicate noble dish and allso you may make balls of Veall & season them with salt peper nutmegs & Currance and so fry them.

Stewed Carp

Ingredients:

1 whole carp
1 pint of water
1 pint of claret
Vinegar, to taste

Mace, to taste
Whole pepper, to taste
Salt, to taste
Lemon, to taste
Sweet herbs, to taste
Onion, to taste

Method: Take a Carpe, open the belly and save the blood, then take a pinte of Water and a pinte of Clarrett Wine, a Little vinegar, some mace and hole Pepper, some salt and a bit of Lemon and a Little Sweet hearbs and some onion. Put these in and Let your Licquor boyle high then put in your Carpe and keep it Close covered. So let it Stew and when it is enough Serve it in some of the same Licquor.

Stewed Haddock or Perch

Ingredients:

3 whole haddocks
Salt, to taste
¼ pound of butter, plus extra for frying
½ a gill, or ⅛ pint of white wine
2 anchovies
Whole pepper, to taste
½ an onion
1 spoonful of ketchup
1 bundle of sweet herbs
Flour

Method: Take three Haddocks, Cut off the Heads, wash & Clean them. Slit them down the Backs, Bone & Cut them in half. Wipe them very dry, put a little Salt on them & Fry them very Crisp in Butter & Drain them. Then take half a Gill of White Wine & as much Water Boyl'd up w'th 2 Anchovies, hole pepper, half an Onionion, a spoone full of Catchup, a fagot of sweet herbs, a Quarter of a pound of Butter rol'd in Flour. Strain the Liquor before you put in to the Haddocks.

Stewed Pigeons with Cabbage

Ingredients:

1 small white cabbage
Milk
6 pigeons
Pepper, to taste
Salt, to taste
1 pint of gravy
Cream or butter, to thicken the gravy
2 yolks

Method: Take a Small White Cabbage, cut it in Small Peces and Just let it Boile in milk & water, then strain the Liquor from it. Then take 6 Pidgons, season them w'th Pepper & Salt in the inside & without. Lay half the Cabbage in a Stewpan. Lay the Pidgons on it & the rest of the Cabbage at the top. Put in a Little of the milk & water in which the Cabbage was boil'd & near a Pint of Gravey. Thicken it up w'th Cream or Butter & the yolks of 2 Eggs.

The Duchess of Portsmouth's Stewed Beef

Ingredients:

1 large rump of beef
Bacon, enough to cover the rump
Salt, to taste
Allspice, to taste
1 spoonful of ale
1 onion, whole
½ pint of white wine
1 spoonful of mango juice

Method: Take a large Rompe of beefe & take of some of the fatt & take the Grate flak bone out of it & then lard it over very deep with Bacon. Then seson it with salt & jeamaco pepper [allspice]. So set it a stewing in a stew pane with one spoonefull of Alle & a whole Oynnon over a jeantell fire for it must stew easely. It must be 12 owers a stirring at least. When it is allmost done add to it halfe a pint of white Wine with one spoonefull of Manggo licker. If you have no mango licker it will do withe out. So sarve it up with rosted sippets.

Turkey à la Daube

Ingredients:

1 turkey
Pepper
Salt
6 garlic cloves, plus extra
Parsley, chopped
Lard
Fatty bacon
1 sprig of thyme
½ pint white wine
Jelly, for serving
Oil and vinegar, for serving

Earthen pot, big enough for the turkey
Larger pot, for boiling water

Method: Draw the Turkey, cut off the Pinions & wipe the inside very Cleane. Rub it w'th peper and Salt & put into it 2 Cloves of Garlick. Cut your Lardings prity large & role them in peper Salt & Chopt parseley & a little Garlick. Y'n Lard your Turkey Cros the Brest & on the Legs then Lap it round round with Slises fat Bacon. Lay it w'th the Brest Downwards in a well Glas'd Deepe Earthen pot that will but Just hold it for the Closer it lyes the better. Put to it 4 Cloves of Garlick, a sprig of thyme & a little parsley with half a pint of white wine. Cover the pot Extreemly close y't no steem can get out then set it in to a pot of Boyle Water. Let it Boyle 4 Houres then take it out & let it stand till it is cold. Serve it up on a napkin & cover it over w'th Jelley. It is to be Eat w'th Oyle & Vinager.

Very Good Wood-Smoked Hams

Ingredients:

Hams
½ peck of common salt
4 oz of saltpetre
4 oz of coarse [muscovado] sugar

Wood, for smoking

Method: Take your hams and beat them very well 'till they are perfectly soft. Let them ly till the next morning, then to each ham take half a peck of common salt, four ounces of salt peter, and four ounces of course sugar. Mix the sugar with the salt very well. Lay some of the salt under and cover them over with the rest. Let them lye twelve hours then turne them and rub them very well and let them lye twelve hours more. Then take them and dry them over wood smoak. They will be ready to eat in six weeks.

Puddings, Pies and Sweets

A sk most people to name a favourite pudding, and with the excpetion of fans of Yorkshire puddings or black puddings, its likely most will opt for a sweet dessert, enjoyed after a main course. But as Peter Brears explains, in the seventeeth and eighteenth centuries it was savoury puddings that were enjoyed and they were eaten in the middle of the day at dinner as a first course. Later in the eighteenth century, sweet puddings became ever more popular, but as Sabine's receipt books show, there was a good mixture of sweet and savoury dishes to be had. Grandma Layer's *Very Good Black Puddings* and an extremely sweet version of *Rice Pudding* are very different tasting examples of this.

Meat-based puddings in this selection include *New College Pudding*, which owes its name to a college of Oxford University. The recipe requires beef suet, as do two recipes for white pudding. Suet is also a feature of a receipt for mince pies, which also requires beef tongue – very different to the popular Christmas treat of today, and indeed a more elaborate version is entitled *Christmas Pyes*, which also includes a very generous dose of fortified wine.

Orange Tarts, *Champagne Goosberries*, *Candied Cowslips* and *Snow Balls* provide some fruity and rather sugary sweets, although sadly the gooseberry receipt doesn't actually contain any champagne.

There is also a recipe for ice cream, which requires ice, allum and bay salt.

Beef Pie in Blood [Beef in Black Pudding]

Ingredients:

1 rump of beef
4 pints of blood
1⅓lb of beef suet
Grated bread
Salt and pepper, to taste
10 yolks
Thyme
Parsley
Pennyroyal
Fried onions

Method: Take a Rump of beef and cut it into thin slices then take 2 quarts of Blood and one and a third pound of Beef Suet, minsed small, and the quantity of 2 rolls of Grated Bread. Then seson the blod & meet, and mix them alltogether with the youlks of 10 eggs. Mix alltogether and let it ligh 24 houers to soak, then bake it in a pastry pan for 5 houer, and when you draw it fill it with Grave. Do not forget to put in some time, parsly, penneroyell and froyed Oynnins.

Barberry Comfits

Ingredients:

Barberries
Treble refined sugar

Method: Take your Barberryes when Stript so from the stalks and Lay 'em upon Chip Sieves before the fire to Rest then Pulp em thro' a very fine Haire Seive, and put to your Pulp such a quantity of Treble Refined Sugar finely scarced as will bring it to such a consistency as to beare roleing on a paper the Shape you would have 'em either for Jumballs [jumbles] or Comfitts.

Batter Pudding

Ingredients:

1 pint of cream
6 yolks
Flour
Sugar
Rose water
Nutmeg

Method: Take a quart of cream, put to it 6 yolks of eggs, take Flour &
mingle it as thick as batter then put some sugar, rose water & nutmeg, &
Butter your dish. You must beat it 'till it goes into the Oven.

Candy Flowers

Ingredients:

Rose water
1 egg white
A bean-sized piece of gum arabic
Flowers, of any edible kind
Double refined sugar
Birching rod, for stirring

Method: Boile a little Rose water with the white of an Egg in a bason.
Work it a little with a birching rod until it be like snow, then let it stand
one houre. Take off the froth, put in the quantity of a bean of gum
arabick and when it is melted and dissolved in water dip your flowers in
then take duble refined sugar being sifted & dust upon them in a clean
platter then sett them in the sunn, turning them now and then. They
will be finely candied as White as any snow. You cannot candy them by
fire or by boiling of Sugar.

Champagne Gooseberries

Ingredients:

1lb of gooseberries (unstoned)
1lb of sugar
½ pint of water

Method: To a pound of gooseberries, before they are stoned, take a pound of sugar and half a pint of water. Boil the sugar and water very well and scum it. Then having your gooseberries stoned and split as little as you can, put them in and cover them. Boil them 'till they cook clear, then put them in to glasses, then strain your liquor upon them. Four ounce pots are better than glasses.

Christmas Pyes

Ingredients:

Tongue
Beef suet, equal to the weight of the tongue
Nutmeg, cloves, mace and sugar to taste
¼lb of raisins
Candied orange and lemon peel
1 citron
Raw lemon peel
Juice of 2 lemons
6 tablespoons of Canary wine [sherry, or fortified wine]
1 handful of currants
Pastry

Method: Boyle a tongue 'till it will peel. When 'tis cold cut it in pieces (leave out the roots) and chop it very small with the weight of very good beef suet. Then put in a little salt and add what nutmeg, cloves, mace and sugar you please. Then stone a quarter of a pound of raisins and cut them very small and stir 'em well into the meat. Then cut some candied orange and lemon peel pretty small with some citron and put in with it a little raw lemon peel shred very small. Squeeze in the juice of two lemons. Put in six spoonsful of Canary or more, and as many currants

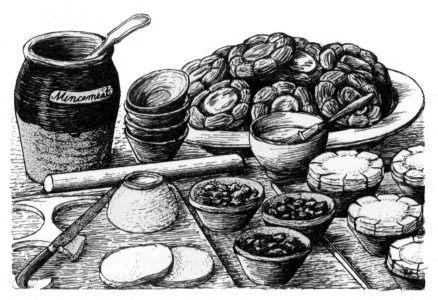

16. Mince Pies by Peter Brears. Based on boiled tongue and suet enriched with dried fruits and sherry, most Georgian mince pies were baked in stoneware patty-pans lined with puff pastry.

as you please. Be sure you stir all well together so that it may have a true mixture. Put the sack in just before you fill your pastry. Bake 'em in a pretty quick oven. When they are almost done the fat will swim on top. When it begins to sink they are ready. If you make your pyes with mutton then boyle a leg (half is enough) and cut it from the sinews and skins, and to every pound of mutton put a pound and a quarter of beef-suet, chopped small and season it to your taste.

Clear Apple Fritters

Ingredients:

Ale or small beer
Batter mixture
Lemon peel
Nutmeg
Salt
Butter
Slices of apple
Hog's lard or beef dripping

Method: Make your Batter w'th Ale or Smallbeer that is not Bitter. Grate in a Lemon peal, if you have it a little nutmeg, & salt, then put in a little oyled Butter to make 'em Crisp. Beat your Batter very well, dip in your slices of Apples & fry them in hogs lard or beef dripping.

Excellent White Puddings

Ingredients:

3 pints of cream
1 pint of new milk
3 grated penny loaves
3 grated nutmegs
1½lb of beef suet
1lb of almonds
Orange flower water
18 eggs
Candied orange and citron peel
Sugar, to taste

Method: Take 3 pints of Cream, one pint of new milk, boyle it & have ready 3 penny Loaves grated, put the Cream to 'em boyleing hot then take 3 nutmegs grated, a pound & a half of beefe Suet, shred very thin, a pound of Almonds, blanch'd & beat very fine with a little Orange Flour water. Put in a Dozen & a half of eggs & some candied Orange & Citron peale. Sweeten it to your Tast [then put into skins and simmer gently].

Flummery

Ingredients:

2 pints of oatmeal
3 pints of water

Method: Take a quart of Oatmeal, put to it 3 pints of Water. Change the water twice a day, the second day strain it thro' a Sieve, & then set it over a soft Fire, keeping it stirring. Let it boyle as least half an hour [then pour into cups and leave to set like jellies].

Fritters

Ingredients:

½ pint of cream
4 eggs
3 egg whites
A little sack (otherwise fortified wine)
Sugar, to taste
Rose water, to taste
1 spoonful of light ale yeast
Apples, as many as needed
Flour

Method: Take half a pint of Creame and 4 Eggs and 3 Whites and a Little Sack, some Suger, Rose Water, and a Spoonfull of the Lightest Ale yeast you can gitt. Pare your Apples and Cut them round and put in flour. To make the batter of the Thickness of Pancakes, stuff and boyle them in Lard. Scrape some suger, so serve them up.

Grandma Layer's Very Good Black Puddings

Ingredients:

Oatmeal (as much as needed)
Hog's blood
Boiled milk
Salt, to taste
Leaf lard
Hog's fat
Grated bread
2 or 3 eggs
Winter savory (otherwise cabbage)
Thyme
Marjoram
Sage
Pennyroyal
Cloves
Mace

Method: Steep some Oatmeal in your Blood & some in milk boyled but first let your Blood stand haveing some salt put in to it when it is new from the hog, till next morning. Then take of the water & put in the Oatmeal being clean, sifted & pick'd. when 'tis steep'd take some of your Leafe of the Hog & boyle it in some milk & put it into the blood & put a good quantity of cut fat in besides, a little grated Bread & 2 or 3 eggs into 2 quarts of pudding a little winter Savory, Thyme, Marjoram, Sage & penny-royall: a good quantity. Season it with Cloves & Mace, fill 'em a little above half full. They must not be prickt. Boyle 'em softly, putting cold water on 'em sometimes to prevent them breaking.

Green Pudding

Ingredients:

1 pint of cream or milk
½ a large bread roll, grated
10 yolks
4 egg whites
2 spoonsful of sack [sherry or fortified wine]
½ a nutmeg, grated
½ a pint of spinach juice
Sugar, to taste
Butter, for greasing

Method: Take a pint of Creme or Milk, half a roll of grated breed, steeped in the youlks of 10 Eggs & 4 whites, 2 spoonefulls of sracke, half a nutmeg grated, halfe a pint of the juse of spenege [spinach] more if it is not greene enough. Sweten it to your taste. So thicken it over the fire then butter your pane & back it.

Ice Cream

Ingredients:

Cream
Double refined sugar

Tin pots, for setting
Pail
Ice
Bay salt
Alum

Method: Sweeten your Cream w'th double refind Sugar and put it into Tin pots & set it into a pail & put some Ice & bay Salt them. Strew some allum upon the ice. Let the Ice be above the pots & in four Houers it will be done.

Lady St Quintin's Dutch Pudding

Ingredients:

2lb of flour
1lb of butter
8 eggs
4 spoonsful of yeast
½ a pint of milk
1lb of currants
Sugarloaf, to taste

Method: Take 2 p'd of Flour, 1 p'd of Butter, 8 Eggs, 4 Spoone fulls of yest. Melt the Butter in half a Pint of Milk, mix 'em well to gether. Let it stand to rise near an Hour then add a p'd of Couranks & a Little lofe Sugar, Grated. An Houre will bake it if it is a hot Oven.

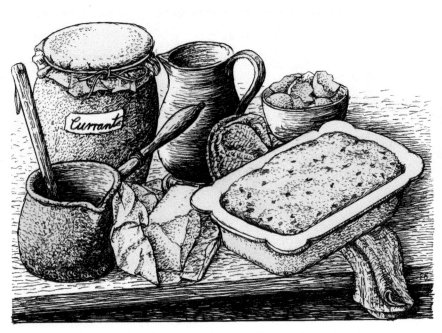

17. Lady St Quintin's Dutch pudding by Peter Brears. From the 1760s, the major Yorkshire potteries were producing both round and rectangular bakers, fine oven-to-table wares ideal for both pies and puddings, such as this Dutch pudding collected from Lady Charlotte St Quintin of Harpham, near Bridlington.

Lady Winn's Mother's Fritters

Ingredients:

8 eggs
1 pint of single cream
A pinch of salt
Cinnamon to taste
Plain flour
4 tablespoons of fortified wine
Some pippins
A good store of hogs fat

Method: Take eight eggs and discard four whites. Beat 'em very well then take a pint of thin cream warmed and put with your eggs. Stir 'em well together with a little salt and cinnamon. Then put in the flour 'till your batter is thick enough. Beat it well and let it stand covered near your fire to rise. Then beat it well again and put in four spoonsful of sack.

Then slice some pippins very thin and put 'em in the batter and take 'em out with a spoon, every slice by itself. Fry 'em with good store of hogs fat, very hot.

Little Baked Puddings

Ingredients:

12 pints of cream
Flour, enough to make a batter
9 yolks
2 egg whites
Butter, for greasing

China cups (ones that will withstand the heat of an oven)

Method: Take a Quart of Cream & stir as much fine flour into it as will make it as thick as for pancakes. Then beat the yolks of nine Eggs & 2 Whites. Put them together & beat them very well. Let the oven be as hot as for Tarts & bake them in China Cups, well Butter'd. They must Stand in Oven three quarters of an hour. Add a Little more flour just before you set them.

To Make a Pudding

Ingredients:

1 pint of cream
4 eggs
One manchet loaf, grated
3 spoonsful of flour
Sack, (fortified wine), to taste
Sugar, to taste
Nutmeg, to taste
Ginger, to taste
Beef suet, enough to thicken the pudding
Butter, to serve
Blanched almonds, to serve

Pudding cloth

Method: Take a pint of cream, 4 Eggs, well betten, & a peney manshett, grated and 3 spoonfull of fine flour. Mix them, season with a Little Sack, sugar & nutmeg, a Little ginger, beef suitt shread very small, as much as will make it fatt, then tye itt in a Cloath & tye it Round. Boyle it in a houre & halfe with the water boyleing before you putt it in. When you serve it up put some beatten butter in the Dish & stick it with almonds cut & sliced & blanched in cold water.

Mince Pies

Ingredients:

1lb of beef tongue
2lb of suet
2lb of currants
½lb of raisins
½lb of candied citron and lemon
½oz of beaten cloves, mace and nutmeg
½ pint of sack (sherry)

Method: Take a neats tongue & boyle it 'till it will peal then slice it & to every pound of minc'd meat put 2 pound of Suet & 2 pound of Currance, one pound of Rasons of the Sun, shred very small & ston'd, half a pound of candied Citron & Lemmon, & almost half an Ounce of Cloves, Mace & Nutmegg beat very fine, half a pint of Sack.

Mrs Cook's Almond Pudding

Ingredients:

1lb of blanched and beaten almonds
Some milk
1lb of grated bread
1lb of sugar
12 yolks
6 egg whites
2 pints of boiled cream
Salt
Nutmeg
1lb of beef marrow

Method: Take a pound of almonds, blanch them and beat them very well. Every now and then add some milk whilst beating to keep them from oyleing. Then mix with them a pound of grated bread, a pound of sugar, twelve eggs, (leave out six whites), a quart of warm creame (having earlier been boyled), as much salt and nutmeg as will season it and a pound of beef marrow.

Mrs Cook's Liver Pudding

Ingredients:

1lb of grated bread
1lb of currants
1½lb of bone marrow and suet
¾lb of sugar
1oz of cinnamon
¼oz of mace
1 pint of grated liver (or as much as desired)
Salt, to taste
6 eggs
6 egg whites
3 pints of cream
Skins, for stuffing (e.g. sausage skins)

Method: Take a pound of grated bread, one pound of currants, a pound and half of marrow and suit [suet] together, cut small. Then take three quarters of a pound of sugar, one ounce of cinnamon, a quarter of an ounce of mace, about a pint of grated liver, or as much as you like, and also some salt. Put all these together. Then take twelve eggs, leave out half the whites, beat them well. Put them to three pints of cream. Make the eggs and creame warme, then put it to the pudding stuffe and stir it well together. So fill them in skins [and simmer gently].

Mrs Cook's Oatmeal Pudding

Ingredients:

1 pint of oatmeal
Milk (enough to steep the oatmeal in)
2 pints of cream
1 loaf of bread, grated
6 eggs
4 yolks
4 or 5 spoonsful of sack, otherwise fortified wine
4 or 5 spoonsful of rosewater
½oz of mace
1lb of sugar
1lb of currants
1lb of beef suet

Skins, for cooking in

Method: Take a pint of oatemeale and steepe it in milke all night, and then boyle it in the milke or creame 'till it is as thick as hasty pudding. Boyle a quart of creame and steep the crumbs of a penny loaf in it, then take ten eggs, leaving out four of the whites, then take 4 or 5 spoonfull of sack, as much rose water, half an ounce of mace, one pound of sugar, as many currants, and beef suit shreaded small. Mingle alltogether and fill them into skins [before simmering gently].

Mrs Eall's Candied Cowslips

Ingredients:

½lb of sugar
Cowslip flowers

Method: Take half a pound Suger & boil it to a candy & when your cowslops are picked pot a bout 6 quarters of the flowers to the suger & let them boil in the suger 'till they be enough then take them out & lay them on a paper and so lay them by for your use.

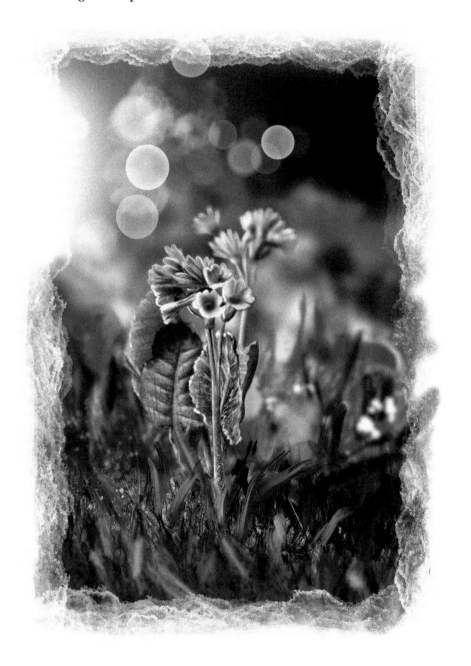

Mrs Ealls' Gooseberry Fool

Ingredients:

4 pints of gooseberries
10 yolks
¾lb of sugar

Method: Take 2 quarce [quarts] of Gousberry, picke thin and put
them into a Skillet with as much water as will cover them. Set them on
a gentill fier to scald & then boyle them tender. They will be an ower
[hour] scalding. Then boyle them up quick & pulpe them throue a hare
sive. Then take 10 yolks of Eggs & beat them very well. Take 3 quarter
of a pounde of Sugar, stir it all to githen with the sugar then put your
Eggs with it & set it on a gentill fier & let it juste boyle up continualy
stirring of it then put it into your dish.

Mrs Wiseman's Pancakes

Ingredients:

6 eggs
Flour, enough to thicken the batter
Sugar, to taste
Nutmeg, to taste
4 spoonsful of Canary wine
Cream, to thin the batter
6 spoonsful of melted butter

Method: Take 6 eggs with the whites, beat 'em very well & thicken
'em very well with Flour & beat 'em 'till they are thin. Sweeten it with
fine Sugar to your Tast & with nutmeg to your Tast, then put to it 4
Spoonfulls of Canary. When these are in make it very thin with Cream.
When you are ready to fry, put in 6 Spoonfulls of Butter, melted, without
water. Beat all well togeth'r. When your pan is warm put in 2 Spoonfulls
& let it run as thin as it can. Then fry 'em without any thing. Your Fire
must be very rash.

New College Pudding

Ingredients:

Loaf of bread
¼lb of beef suet
½ a nutmeg
2 eggs
Currants, to taste
Sugar, to taste
Flour, for dusting your hands

Method: Grate a toopeny Loaf, a quarter of a pound of beef suet, half a Nutmegg grated, 2 Eggs well beat, a few Currants. Mix them all together with Shuger to your tast. Flour your hands & rowl them up in the Shape of an egg. Fling then into boyling hot water. When they Rise they are enough.

Orange Tarts

Ingredients:

12 Seville oranges
Pastry for tart bases (made using any preferred recipe)
2lb of sugar
Lemon juice, if needed

Method: Take 12 of the best Sevill Oranges, pare off the Rines as thin as you can. When par'd put 'em into a pan of fair water as you pare 'em, then cut 'em in two & squeeze out all the Juce still throwing 'em into fair Water as you do 'em. Then take out all the Seeds from the Juce & put 'em into half a pint of water & let 'em stand till you have made your Tarts. Then take your Orang peals & boyle 'em in a pot of Water & when they have boyl'd two hours pour that water from 'em & boyle 'em in another 'till they are very tender then take 'em off the Fire & take the Skinney part all out, still puting 'em into cold water as you do 'em. Then take your Oranges & cut 'em into thin slices, still puting 'em into fresh Water & when they are all slic'd take 'em out of the Water & put 'em into a Cullender for draining. Then fit your Tarts & take the Juce &

the Water where the Seeds are (which will be a sort of Jelly) & strain 'em out together & put 4 or 5 Spoonfulls of the Juce into every Tart. 2 pound of Sugar will serve your 12 Oranges & 12 Oranges will make 12 Tarts. It must be fine Sugar. Half an hour or thereabouts bakes 'em. Note: if your Oranges will not afford Juce enough, you may take the Juce of a Lemmon mixt with a little Water & supply your Tarts with that Liquor.

Rice Pudding

Ingredients:

6oz of powdered rice
2 pints of milk
½lb of butter
6 eggs
½ a nutmeg
Sack (otherwise fortified wine), to taste
Sugar, to taste
Sugar paste, to garnish
Citron and lemon peel, to garnish

Method: Take 6 ounces of Rice in Powder & boyle it in a quart of milk, keeping it stirring 'till it is very thick. Then take it off the Fire and stirr in half a pound of Butter, 6 very well beaten Eggs, halfe a sliced nutmegg, sack & sugar to your Taste. Garnish the Dish with Sugar Paste and lay on as much Citron & Lemon peel as you please.

Marrow Pudding

Ingredients:

2 pints of cream
½lb of blanched almonds
Canary wine, to taste
Sugar, to taste
½lb of raisins
½lb of brisket
Marrow from two bones
Puff pastry

Method: Take a quart of Cream & boyle it & when 'tis half cold put to it half a pound of Almonds blanch'd & pounded in a mortar with a little Canary & Sugar, half a pound of Resons ston'd & half a pound of Brisket cut in Slices with the marrow of two Bones then lay some marrow, Brisket & Resons on the bottom of your Dish & put on it some of the Cream. Do this 3 or 4 times 'till your Dish is full, then garnish your Dish with Puff-pastry.

Sago Pudding

Ingredients:

2 pints of milk
1 pint of water
5 spoonsful of sago

Method: Take a pint of Milk & as much Water & put to 'em 5 Spoonfulls of Sago when 'tis wash'd. Boyle it together 'till it is thick and then put in a pint more of milk & boyle it.

Snow Balls

Ingredients:

Stewed apples
Thin tart crust (made to any favoured recipe)
Icing (made to any favoured recipe)

Method: Take your Apples Stew'd whole as for the table. Cover them with thin tart Crust. Make them as round as you can. Set them into the Oven 'till the Paste is enough, then take them out & ice them so set them in again 'till the Iceing is harden'd. So send them to Table Hot or Cold which you chuse.

Spanish Pap

Ingredients:

3 yolks
3 spoonsful of rice flour
3 spoonsful of sugar
1 pint of cream
Snow cream, (or whipped cream), to serve

China cups, to serve

Method: Take the yolkes of 3 eggs, 3 Spoonfulls of Rice flour, 3 Spoonfulls of Sugar, a pint of cream. Set all these over a Fire keeping 'em stirring 'till they are thick enough, then take it off & serve it up in China Cups or Basons w'th Snow Cream.

Sugar of Red Roses

Ingredients:

1oz of red rose leaves
1 of sugar
Juice of 1 lemon
Gum tragacanth
Rose water

Method: Take one ounce of Red Rose leaves, the white being cut off and pulverized very fine then take one pound of loaf sugar finely powdered. Mix them well together in a marbill morter then take the Juce of a Lemon newly squeezed and a Little gumm adragant [gum tragacanth] dissolved in Rose water and strained and so beate them into a past by mixing a little of the Juce and a Little of the gumm at a time and so form them into what forms you Please.

Tansy Pudding

Ingredients:

2 pints of cream
1 small bread roll, grated
3 Naples biscuits
14 yolks
8 egg whites
½ nutmeg
Mace, to taste
½lb of sugar
¼ pint of sack, otherwise fortified wine
½ pint of spinach juice
Salt, to taste
Sweet butter, for frying

Method: Take a quart of cream, boyle it, put to it a penny-loafe grated & 3 Naples bisket. Cover it close 'till it is cold. Beat 14 eggs, leave out 6 whites. Then take half a nutmegg, boyle some mace in the Cream, half a pound of Sugar, a quart'r of a pint of Sack, half a pint of Spinnage-juice, a little salt. Beat all these well together then fry it w'th sweet Butter. Let it stand a quart'r of an hour over a soft Fire then serve it up.

White Puddings

Ingredients:

2 roasted capons, free range
1lb bacon fat
Thyme, to taste
Pennyroyal, to taste
1 hot onion, chopped
Pepper, to taste
Salt, to taste
Cloves, to taste
Mace, to taste
Nutmeg, to taste
2 white loaves, made into breadcrumbs

12 yolks
2 pints of cream
Sheep guts, or other type of skin
Milk, for boiling

Method: Take all the brown and flesh of a couple of roasted Capons. Mince the flesh very small with the marrow of the bones and a pound of the fat of the best Bacon you can get, laid in water before you use it. Add thime, penyroyall, a hot onyon chopt very small, peper, salt, cloves, mace and nutmegs with the crumbs of 2 white Loves and the yolks of 12 Eggs and a quart of Cream mix't all together and fill your sheeps guts, being ready, therewith. Let them boyle in milk and water for half an hour. When cold, cut them in half and broil [grill] them upon paper.

Soups, Sauces and Sides

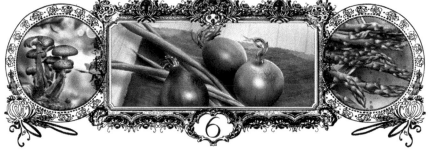

6

This shorter selection contains a recipe simply entitled *Soup*. If ever a title didn't do justice to the receipt, this is it. An epic recipe, not untypical of the period, includes twenty ingredients ranging from a piece of lean beef to a whole duck or chicken, with spinach, sorrel, shallots, sweet and mixed herbs, anchovies and even white wine thrown in to keep adding to the flavour. Larger households, and they didn't get very much grander than Nostell, had the space to keep vast stocks of ingredients. A family recipe for onion soup, another of K. Winn's contributions to the receipt books, contained twelve 'large' onions, veal, mutton and a gallon of water. Big cooking pots and enourmous kitchens might be a bonus if attempting either of these!

This section also includes a dressing (for a mock turtle), a sauce (for fish), and cauliflower, artichoke and cucumber dishes that could be served today as sides or starters. There's also a pretty easy receipt for homemade mustard.

Artichoke Florentine

Ingredients:

Globe Artichokes
Whole pepper
Mace
The marrow of 2 large bones
6 egg yolks, hard boiled
Candied orange and citrus
Green gooseberries or grapes
Vinegar
Sugar
Eggs

Method: First boyle your Heartychokes, then take as many Bottoms as will cover the dish, then throw in a little whole pepper & mace with the marrow of 2 large bones, the yolkes of 6 eggs boyld hard & cut small with some candied orange & Citron. And when you have 'em, green Goosberries or Grapes to place ab't the edges. Then bake it & when it comes out of the Oven, make a Cawdle of Vineg'r, sug'r & eggs & put into the Dish.

Cauliflower au Galantine

Ingredients:

2lb of a leg of veal, to be boiled in liquor
Salt and pepper, to taste
Mace
1 sweetbread
Boiled truffles and morels
Forcemeat balls
1 cauliflower, plus extra pieces
Thick white gravy

Method: Take 2 Pound of a Leg of Veal, boill it in liquor 'till enough then pound it in a marble mortar with a little of the liquor it was Boil'd in to make it a stiff Paste. Season it to your taste with Salt, Pepper &

mace, then lay it in your Dish & make it about an Inch high at the sides, then Bake it a Little, then have ready a sweet Bread boil'd & cut in Pieces, some Truffles and Morrels Boiled, some small force meat balls & a few pieces of Coliflower. Toss them all up in a thick white Gravy & put them into your Crust, then have ready a coliflower Lightly Boiled & Pul'd to Pieces as for pickling & put it at the top with the Flower Part upwards as Close as if it was one entire Flower then set it in the Oven 'till you think the Meat is enough. So serve it up.

Dressing for an English Turtle

Ingredients:

1 calf's head
Flour
Cayenne pepper, to taste
Mace, to taste
Nutmegs, to taste
Salt, to taste
1 pint of Madeira wine
Veal gravy
Yolks of hard boiled eggs
Forcemeat balls
Lemon slices, to garnish

Method: Take a Calves head w'th the Skin on. Scald the Hair off & wash it clean, then cut it in pieces & dust some flour on to it. Season w'th Coyan Peper, mace, nutmegs & salt. Put the whole in to a Pitcher w'th one full pint of Madeira wine & the quantity of Vealgravy that will cover it. Lay at the top of your Pitcher some yolks of hard Eggs and as many forsmeat balls as you can till the pitcher is full, then lye a paper & Blader on the Top & set it in to the Oven where it must remain four Hours & serve it up w'th a Garnish of Slic'd Lemon only.

Fish Sauce

Ingredients:

Mace, to taste
Cloves, to taste
Whole peppercorns, to taste
A bundle of sweet herbs
Spring water
Butter, to taste
1 anchovy
1 onion
1 pint of shrimps
Oysters, to taste

Method: Take a little Mace, Cloves, whole pepp'r, and a bundle of sweet herbs. Boyle all these in Spring water 'till it tast well, then put it into a Sauce pan & as much Butter as you think fit, one Anchovie, 1 Oynion. While this is stewing put in a pint of Shrimps & as many Oysters if you please.

French Beans with Cream

Ingredients:

Beans
Salt, to taste
Lumps of butter
1 bunch of sweet herbs
Butter
Flour
Sugar, to taste
Cream, to taste

Method: Take your Beans, cut them in thin Long Slices, wash them in hot water & Salt. Put them in a Cullender to Draine then put them in a Stewpan with some Lumps of Butter & a Bunch of Sweet Hearbs. Set them on the fire, toss them up, shake in a little flour, moisten them w'th boyleing water as you see occasion. Season with salt and a little bit of sugar. Let them stew & when are ready to be serv'd up put in a little cream. Serve them up hot for Entermessis [appetizers].

How to Prepare Sparagrass

Ingredients:

Bundle of asparagus
Fresh mint
Cream
Pepper, to taste
Salt, to taste
Nutmeg, to taste
1 yolk (optional)

Method: Take small Sparagrass about the bigness of a Quill and cut them in small square peaces. Putt mint in to it and boyle it together as you please, 'till they are soft. Strain them out of the water. Take cream and put to them and heat it together then season it with peper, salt and nutmeg to your Tast. If it is not Thick Enuff put yolk of a Egg in to it.

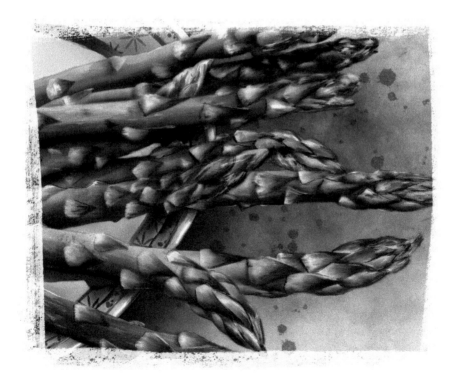

Morels à la Crème

Ingredients:

Morels
Butter
Pepper
Salt
Parsley
Thyme
Veal broth
3 or 4 yolks
¼ of a pint of cream

Method: Take off the Stalks, cut them in three or four pieces if they are large ones. Wash them in severall waters very clean. Put them into a stewpan w'th Butter, Pepper, Salt, parsley & Thyme. Stew all these over the fire till most of the Butter is washed. You must ad Veal broth to stew, the yolks of 3 or 4 Eggs & a quarter of a pint of Cream, then stew them up. You may do moshrooms the same way.

Mrs K. Winn's Onion Soup

Ingredients:

2lb of veal
2lb of mutton
1 gallon of water
1 French roll
12 large onions
Butter, for frying
Salt and pepper, to taste

Method: Take 2 pd of Veal and 2 pd of mutton. Boil them in a galon of Water 'till it comes to 2 Quarts then Strain it & take off all the fat, then toast the uper & under Crust of a french Role very brown. Put it in to the Broath. Slise 12 large onions and fry them in Butter 'till they are very brown. Put them in the broath and boil them in the broth half an Houer. Add peper & Salt to your tast and so serve it up.

Mustard

Ingredients:

Mustard seed
White wine vinegar
Horseradish
Sugar

Method: Dry the [mustard] seed in an Oven. Beat it well in a morter and seave it through a fine sive. Take the flour thereof and put to it a Quantety of the best white wine vinegar. Put into your vinegar a day before you use it a little horseredish and when you have mix't the vinegar with the flour of the mustard seed put to it a little peece of fine loaf shugar and cover it close in a pot. Let it sit foure or five dayes before you use it.

Pistachio Cream for Chicken

Ingredients:

2 pints of cream
Sugar
¼lb of pistachios, well pounded
2 chicken gizzards
Spinach juice (optional)

Method: Take a Quart of Cream & put to it a small quantity of Sugar. Let it Boyl then take a Quarter of a lb of Pistacha, let them be well pounded, then take a Couple of the Gisards of a fowl that is the inside skin. Wash it well & cut it small. Put it in to a Cup & put to it some of the Boyald Cream, luke warm. Set it near the fire till it cums then strain it and then put in your Pastatios & set it near the Fire again cover'd up close & it will become thick. Then set it to coole but mind that your Dish stands level. If you would have it greener than the pistachios will make it, add a little Juise of spinnage.

Regalia of Cucumbers

Ingredients:

12 cucumbers
Flour, for dusting, plus enough to thicken the sauce
⅛ of a pint of claret
½ a pint of gravy
Salt, to taste
Pepper, to taste
Cloves, to taste
Mace, to taste
Nutmeg, to taste
Butter, to taste

Lamb, mutton or veal, to serve

Method: Take 12 Cowcumbers & Slice them. Put them in a Clean Cource Cloath. Beat & Squeeze them 'till dry then Flour & Fry them brown. Put to them half a Quarter of a Pint of Claret, half a pint of Gravy, a little salt, pepper, cloves, mace & nutmeg, a little Butter, thickned w'th Flour. Toss it up. They are Sause for Lamb or Mutton, also for Veal Cutlets.

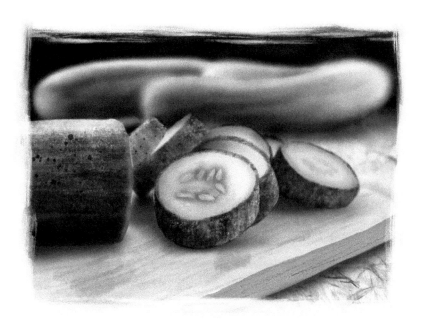

Soup

Ingredients:

1 piece of lean beef
1 knuckle of veal
1 scrag end of a neck of mutton
Salt, to taste
1 bunch of sweet herbs
3 or 4 shallots
Whole pepper, to taste
1 race of ginger
1 nutmeg, sliced
2 or 3 handfuls of spinach
1 or 2 handfuls of sorrel
Mixed herbs, to taste
5 or 6 ox palates
3 or 4 sheeps' tongues, boiled and sliced
2 or 3 veal sweetbreads
1 whole duck or chicken, to serve
2 small white bread buns, cut into pieces
1 pint of white wine
3 or 4 anchovies
Shredded lemon, to serve

Deep dish, to serve

Method: Take a piece of lean beef, that is fit for gravy with a Knuckle of Veal & the Crag end of a neck of Mutton & put it into a pot with more water than will cover it & a little Salt. When it boyles skim it clean & put to it a Bunch of Sweet herbs with 3 or 4 Shellots, a little whole pepper, a race of Ginger & a nutmegg slic'd. Let this boyle on a Soft fire 'till tis boyl'd all to pieces then straine it & take off all the fat & put it into the pot again & put to it 2 or 3 handfulls of Spinnage, a handfull or two of Sorrell, a few of all sorts of Herbs, 5 or 6 Ox-pallats, 3 or 4 Sheeps tongues being boyl'd tender & cut into little slices and 2 or 3 Veal Sweet-breads cut into bits. Put to it a Duck or Pullet & 2 penny white loavs cut into little bits with a pint of White wine. Let these boyle together almost an hour. Put in 3 or 4 Anchovies & put it in a deep dish with the Duck in the middle & garnish with Shred Lemmon.

Wines, Spirits, Vinegars and Waters

This final selection covers some of the many beverages found in the receipt books, and also a couple of vinegars. Some of the receipts for alcoholic drinks involve distilling. This is illegal in the UK without a distiller's licence and obviously rather dangerous without the required knowledge and experience to carry it out. Therefore these receipts shouldn't be attempted. The law does not prevent beer and wine making and these drinks were as popular then as now, wine especially so within the circles that Sabine Winn's husband, Sir Rowland, craved to mix.

The first receipt below, for *Boxed Wine*, is interesting in that it was to be made in a 'Chocolote pot', an oranate, tall vessel, a bit like an elaborate teapot. Chocolate was a drink that had only become popular in England during the previous century, when chocolate and coffee houses reached the capital in the 1650s. The first coffee house opened in Cornhill in 1652, followed in 1657 by the very first chocolate house, which opened near Bishopgate. Other wines below include *Cherry Wine*, requiring just cherries and sugar to make it, plus receipts, among others, for cowslip, elder, sage, sycamore and even quince wine!

Brandy was a poplar liquor in Sabine Winn's time. You might imagine that raspberry and lemon brandies are more likely to be found on a stall at a modern-day food festival or farmer's market than in the receipt books but these fruits are represented in the two brandies chosen for inclusion below.

K. Winn's final contribution is a receipt for *Usquebaugh*, which is another way of saying Irish whiskey, the full title being *Usquebaugh, as given to Mrs K. Winn by a Gentleman who brought it out of Ireland.* You're probably going to have to imagine the taste, but what a variety of flavours to be had: nutmeg, mace, cinnamon, cloves, liquorice, coriander seeds, aniseed, ginger, honey, treacle and saffron all being mixed into malt whiskey, French brandy or cider!

There are also receipts for several aromatic waters: elder, contributed by Lady Sunderland; and orange and cinnamon being favourite flavours. There is also a milk water made originally for Sir Rowland Winn. Depending on when the receipt was written, it would have been given either to Sabine's husband, who died in 1785, or her son, of the same name and title, who was born a decade before his father's death. It had been prepared by the apothecary Charles Mason, and contains, among other things, meadowsweet, mint, balm and blessed thistle, and was probably given for an upset stomach. The next chapter of this book provides many remedies that might have helped such a complaint.

Boxed Wine

Ingredients:

1 pint of strong white wine, plus extra
½ a pint of water
3 eggs
Sugar
Juice of 1½ half lemons

Method: Take a pint of Strong white wine & half a pint of water. Let them boyl. Then beat 3 Eggs with some Shuger & a little wine, then let the wine be all most cold & mix them together & Strain it through a hare seive. Put it into a Chocolate pot & set it over the fire, stirring it all the while. When you think it is ready take it off & put to it the Jus of a Lemmon & a half, & Shuger as you please and Mill it like Chocolate.

Cherry Wine

Ingredients:

Cherries
¼lb of sugar for every gallon of cherry juice

Method: Stalk your Cherries, than break 'em with your hands in a Tub very well, let 'em stand so all night cover'd. The next day strain it & put the wine into a Rundlet. To every Gallon of the Juice put a quart'r of a pound of Sugar & bung it up well. Let it stand a Month, then draw it out into Bottles, stop 'em very close & set 'em very cool.

Cinnamon Water

Ingredients:

4 pints of brandy
4 pints of running water
4oz of cinnamon

Method: Put to 2 quarts of Brandy 2 of running water & four Ounces of Cinnamon. Steep it one day & a night, close stop'd, then distill in a cold-still w'th a gentle fire & draw it as long as you like the taste.

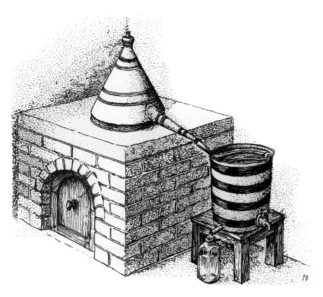

18. Cinnamon water by Peter Brears. To distil alcoholic and medicinal 'waters', many ladies used a 'cold still'. This had the 'cucurbit' or boiler set within a masonry stove, over which was fitted a conical 'alembic' that collected the steam and the condensed liquid that formed inside. These were fed into a spiral tube or 'worm' in a tub of water that cooled them before they dropped into a bottle.

Cowslip Wine

Ingredients:

Water
Sugar (2lb for every gallon of water)
Cowslips: ½ bushel for every four gallons of water
4 lemons (juice of 4 and peel of ½ a lemon)
Slice of toast with yeast spread on it

Method: To every Gallon of Water put 2 pound of Sugar, & to every 4 Gallons half a Bushell of pickt Cowslips or more. Boyle your Water & Sugar for 3 quarter of an Hour, & scum it, bruise your Cowslips a little, put 'em into an earthen pot & pour your Water & Sugar scolding hot upon 'em. Stir 'em & cover 'em up close & let 'em stand 2 dayes, then strain 'em out & put the liquor into the same pott again. Take 4 good Lemmons, strain the Juce of 'em into the Wine, put half a Lemmon-peal into it, spread a Toast over with yest, put it into it, cover it up close & warm one night, then take out the Toast, & put the Liquor into a Vessell. Let it stand 7 or 8 Weeks, then bottle it off.

Duchess of Norfolk's Punch

Ingredients:

8 lemons
8 oranges
1 gallon of brandy
2 gallons of fair water
4lb of fine sugar
8 egg whites

1 barrel

Method: Take the paring of eight lemons and as many oranges, pared very thin. Steep 'em in a gallon of brandy and keep closed for 24 hours. Then take two gallons of fair water (or something more if you like it smaller). Add four pound of fine sugar and clarify it while it boils with the whites of eight eggs. Let it boil a quarter of an hour and skim it very well. Let it stand 'till 'tis cold then strain the brandy from the parings and mix it with the clarified water and put in the juice of the lemons and oranges, which were pared. Then put it in a barrel, stop it close for three months and then bottle it. If it does not come fine in that time, keep it longer in the barrel.

Elder Wine

Ingredients:

20lb of Malaga Raisins
40 pints of spring water
6 pints of elderberry syrup:
    A 'great quantity' of ripe elderberries
    1lb of sugar for every 2 pints of juice

Method: Take 20 pounds of Mallaga raisons, pick them from the stalks, chap them very small and put them into a tub with 20 quarts of Spring water and let them stand ten dayes, stiring them twice a day with a stick, then straine the liquor out from the raisons very hard, and put to the liquor six pints of the syrup of elder berries. Stop it very close in a vessell, let it stand six weeks before you bottle it, or longer. If it is not fine, it will keep three years.

How to make the syrup of elder for the wine: take a great quantity of elder berries full ripe, put them into a Jug, set them into a kettle of boyling water, and as they infuse draine the liquor from them, and to every quart of Juce add a pound of Sugar. Boyle them together as you doe for other syrup.

Elderflower Vinegar

Ingredients:

1 vessel of vinegar
Elderflowers

Method: You must have a vessel of vinegar reddy of what quantity you please and when the Elder flowers are full ripe they must be pickt cleane from the stalks but after ward you must spread them a broad that they may be dry before you put them into the vinegar. After the flowers are in stop up your vessell verry close. Wee used to make half a keggs head at a time and when up to put in a bushell of flower after they are pickt.

Elderflower Wine

Ingredients:

6 gallons of water
10lb of sugar
6lb of raisins
¼ of a peck of elderflowers
6 spoonsful of lemon syrup
4 spoonsful of good ale yeast

Method: Take 6 gallons of Water, ten pounds of suger, 6 pounds of Rasons. Boyle them together for an houer. The flowers of the Elder must be to the quantity of a quarter of a peck. Put them in when the Liquour is very cold. The next day put in 6 spoonefulls of syrup of lemons & 4 of good Alle yeast and 2 days after put it into a Vessell. It must be filled up with Liquor at 6 months and bottall it. If fine, it will not come to the right taste under a twelve month time.

Gooseberry Wine

Ingredients:

1 peck of ripe gooseberries
8 pints of white wine
2 pints of Rhenish wine
Sugar, to taste

Method: Take a peck of goosberries through ripe, bruse them well and put them in a pitcher then put to them 4 quarts of white wine & 1 quart of Renish & stir them very well together & stop them cloase when thay have stood three hours runn it through a flanning bagg [flannel bag] puting back the first till it runns clear, and then boyle it with a lump of Loafe sugar. It will keep all the year.

Lady Strickland's Strong Mead

Ingredients:

7 pints of water
2 pints of honey
6 egg whites
Yeast, spread on toast
Lemon slices

Method: To every 3 Quarts of water one Quart of Honey. Stir them well together. Set them on the Fire and when it is near boyling put in the whites of 6 Eggs, well beaten, in a Pint of water. Dash down the scum 3 times before you take it off. Boyl it one Hower or more, & when it is almost colde set on a little [yeast] spread on a tost [toast] & Slises of Lemon, Less or more as you like the tost.

Lady Sunderland's Elder Water

Ingredients:

1 gallon of crushed elderberries
1 pint of cask ale

Method: Take Elder Berries when thay are full ripe and Pick them from the stalks and mash them well together & put them into a great Earthen pot but not full & to every Gallon a pint of good cask & stirr it well together. Then Lett it stand & Work 2 or 3 dayes Stirring it well with a Stick every day then put it into a Limbeck [otherwise an alembic] and so draw it off.

Lady Winn's Mother's Gooseberry Wine

Ingredients:

1 gallon of very ripe gooseberries
1 gallon of water
2lb of fine sugar

Method: Take a Gallon of very ripe Goosberries, bruise 'em in a Mortar, & to every Gallon of Gooseberries put a Gallon of Water &

let 'em stand 2 days & nights, stirring 2 or 3 times a day. Strain it thro' a Hair bag, let it stand & settle a day & night & to every Gallon of clear Juice put 2 p'd of fine Sug'r. Let it work in a Vessell that is quite full & when 'tis clear & very fine bottle it off. Corke it but loosely 3 or 4 dayes.

Lemon Brandy

Ingredients:

3 pints of your favourite brandy
Peel of 10 lemons
½lb of sugar
1 pint of water

Bottles

Method: Take 3 pints of Brandy. Take the peale of 10 Leamonse, cut as thine as possebell. Let it stande 2 dayse then take half a pound of Lofe Suger & a pynt of water. Make it intow a Syrup, boyle and sieve into the bottells. Orange Brandy is made the same way.

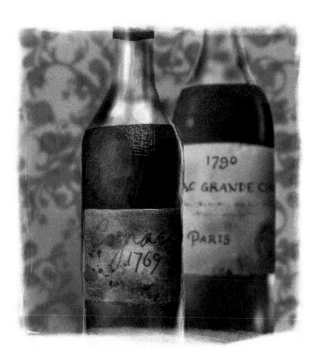

Mrs Eall's Mead

Ingredients:

1 gallon of water
1 pint of honey
Spices, to taste
½ pint of good yeast

Method: To every galon of water take a pint of hony, som spice to your tast. Set it on the fier & let it boyl a bout an houer then so take it off & let it stand a Coling & when it is almost Cold put to it half a pint of good yeast & then put it in to your vessell. Let it stand 10 days then botel it off.

Orange Wine

Ingredients:

3 gallons of water
6lb of sugar
2 egg whites
100 Seville oranges
Yeast

Method: Take three gallons of water and six pounds of sugar. Boyle 'em half an hour, then scum it. Then clarifye it with the whites of two eggs and when 'tis cool put in the juice and outward rinds of a quart of a hundred Seville oranges. Work it with yeast and let it work for twenty-eight hours in an open tub. Then strain it and put it into a vessel and in a fortnight's time draw it off.

Another Orange Wine

Ingredients:

6 gallons of water
12lb of sugar
6 egg whites
50 oranges

6 spoonsful of wine yeast
2 pints of sack, otherwise fortified wine

Barrel for wine making
Bottles

Method: Take 6 gallons of Water, 12 pounde of Suger, the white of 6 Eggs, well beaten. Boyle it an Hour & scum it well. Pare 50 Orranges as thine as you can & power the licker boyling hot upon your peels. Let it stand 'till it is allmost cold, then add in 6 spoonefuls of yeast, the juce of the Orranges straned through a sive, and a quart of sacke. Let it worke 48 hours beatting it in sometimes, then put it into a barrell & let it stand 3 weeks. Then if it be cleen bottell it.

Quince Wine

Ingredients:

4lb of quinces, peeled and cored
1 gallon of spring water
3lb of sugar

Fermentation vessel
Bottles

Method: Take 4 pound of Quinse parred & corr'd. Beat & bruse them. Put them to a Gallond of spring watter & let them be infused 24 hours then strain them to which Lickker. Put 3 pound of Shuger, stir it well 'till all the Shuger be melted then put it into a vissill. Let it stand 3 months to fine & then Bottle it.

Note: if the above quantity yields too little wine, try 12 pound of Quinse & 3 Gallons of watter with 10 pound of Shuger.

Raspberry Brandy

Ingredients:

2 pints of brandy
3 pints of raspberries
Sugar, to taste

Earthen pot
Bottles

Method: To a quart of Brandy take 3 pints of Rasberries. Bruise 'em a little, put 'em into the Brandy in an Earthen pot close cover'd & let 'em stand a Week stirring 'em now & then. Strain 'em throw a Hair Sieve & sweeten it to your Tast with fine Sugar & let it stand a week to settle then Bottle it & if it is not fine draw it into fresh Bottles.

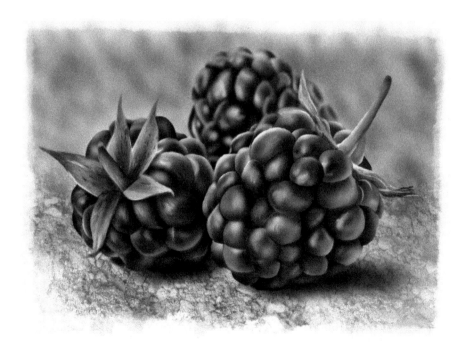

Right Red Dutch Currant Wine

Ingredients:

½ a gallon of currant juice
½ a gallon of boiled water
1lb of double refined sugar
Egg whites, for clarifying
1 piece of loaf sugar per bottle

Barrel
Bottles

Method: Let your Currants hang on the Trees 6 or 7 weeks after they red, then take the same quantity of water, boyle the water with a pound of double refin'd Sug'r to a Gallon of your Wine when mix't with your Water & when the water is cold mix it with your Juice, & clarifye it with the whites of eggs. This will make it indifferent clear. So draw it out at a tap into a Barrell & in a month you may bottle it off, putting a peice of Loafe Sug'r into each Bottle. It will be fit to drink in 7 or 8 weeks.

Sage Wine

Ingredients:

6 gallons of spring water
24lb of Malaga raisins
½ bushel of sage
1 lump of sugar per bottle

Bottles

Method: Take 6 Gallons of Spring water. Let it boyle ab't an hour & have ready 24 po'd of Mallage Resons pick't & shred small, then put 'em into a Tub & pour the water boyleing hot on 'em. At the same time put in almost half a Bushell of the best Sage, pick't & shred small. Stir in well together once every day, then strain it as dry as you can & let the Vessell be full. When 'tis clear, bottle it off, puting in a Lump of Sug'r into every Bottle.

Shrub

Ingredients:

4 pints of brandy
2 pints of Rhenish wine
6 lemons (saving 5 of the rinds)
2 pints of water
2½lb of sugar

Stone or earthen jugs, with stoppers or lids
Bottles

Method: Take 2 quarts of Brandy, 1 quart of Rhenish wine, 6 Lemmons, 5 of the Rines, then take off all the white of the Lemmons & slice the Lemmons takeing out the Seeds, 1 quart of water, 2 pound & half of the best loafe Sugar broaken into Lumps. Put all these into a Stone or earthen Jug & stop it down close. Stir it once a day for 4 or 5 dayes then let it run thro' a Sieve, then bottle it into large bottles. Let it stand a Fortight & put it into pints. This will keep 4 or 5 years & the Older the better.

Sir Rowland Winn's Milk Water
(as made by Mr Charles Mason, the apothecary)

Ingredients:

Three handfuls of:
    Meadowsweet
    Mint
    Balm
Two handfuls of:
    Cardo santo, otherwise blessed thistle
    Goat's rue
    Roman wormwood
One handful of:
    Angelica
    Teucrium scordium, otherwise water germander
    Borage
Four gallons of new milk

Still

Method: Take Meadowsweete, Mint and Balm, of Eache 3 handfulls, Cardos, Goats Rue, and Roman Wormwood, of each 2 handfulls, Angelico, Scordium [water germander], Borage, Each one handful. Cut & mix alltogether and with 4 Gallons of new milke. Distill it in a cold still. This is the milke Water S'r Rowland Winn likes given by Mr Charles Mason Apoticary

Smyrna Wine

Ingredients:

150 raisins
Hogshead of water

A barrel

Method: To a Hundred & a half of Smirna Currants put half a Hogshead of Raw Water (River Water if near, any if not) the softest you can & put them into a Tub & Stir twice a Day. To make it work, let it work three weeks or 'till the sweetness of the Currants is Gone off. Sometimes it will be gone of in a fortnight, if the Weather be warm it works quicker. Let it stand two or three Days Without stiring it before you Draw it off, to Let the Currants Settle. Put the Liquor into a Barrell & lay a Paper over the Bung hole for a Fortnight or three Weeks then Clay it up very Close. It should stand half a year Before you Bottle it. If it is not fine then let it stand 'till it is. Cover the Tub whilst it works. March or April is the Best time to make it.

Strong Mead

Ingredients:

3 gallons of water
8 pints of honey
4 egg whites
1oz of ginger, nutmeg and cloves
White toast dipped in ale yeast

Method: Take 3 Gallons of Water & warm it, then put in 4 quarts of Honey & dissolve it well then take the Whites of 4 eggs well beaten & put into the Water & Honey, & with a clean whisk beat 'em altogether then boyle it & as the skim ariseth take it clean off & to every 6 gallons of mead you must allow two to be boyl'd away. Put to it one ounce of Ginger, nutmeggs & cloves grosely cut, & when 'tis boyl'd enough pour it off into severall vessels & when tis almost cold put it all into one Tub & put to it a white Toast dipt in Ale yest & let it work 24 hours being close cover'd up. Tun it next day & when it has done working, bung it close. But if it does not work in a day or two stop it up & in 3 or 4 months time you may drink of it. But 'tis generally kept a year before us'd. Be sure to measure the water & Honey in the same pot.

Sycamore Wine

Ingredients:

1 gallon of sycamore tree liquor
2lb of powdered sugar
Ale yeast
2lb of raisins for every 5 gallons of wine
Isinglass
½ pint of brandy

Tree tapping equipment
Barrel smoked with brimstone

Method: Early in the mounth of March tap the Trees, keep the Rain from mixing w'th the Liquor as much as possible. To a Galon of the Liquor put 2 pound of powder Sugar. Boyle it well & scum it. Put it in a Tub & when it is luke warme put on a little new ale yeast. Let it worke 5 or 6 days stiring it twice a day. When you tun it add 2 pound of Reasons, chop't a Little, to every 5 galons & 2 peniworth of Ising Glas & about half a pint of Brandy. Let it stand 'till Micklemas. The Barrill should be Smok'd w'th Brimstone. The Liquor will only run when the Sun Shines.

Usquebaugh, as given to Mrs K. Winn by a Gentleman who brought it out of Ireland

Ingredients:

10 gallons of oat malt whiskey, French brandy or cider spirit
½oz of nutmeg
½oz of mace
½oz of cinnamon
½oz of cloves
1 stick of liquorice
½lb of coriander seeds
1oz of aniseed
1oz of cardamom
1oz of ginger
5lb of honey
2½lb of treacle
10oz of saffron
10lb of loaf sugar

Method: To Tenn Gallons of the finest Spirit (which in Ireland is generally drawne from Oatemalt, or French Brandy if you can't get it but a good Cyder Spirit will do very well) take nutmegs, Mace, Synamon & Cloves of each halfe an Ounce. Stick liquorish halfe a pound, Cariander Seeds, Anniseeds Cardrinum & Ginger of each one Oz To every Gallon there must be honey halfe a pound. Treacle a quarter of a pound, Safron one ounce. (The more Treakle the less Saffron.) Loafe Suger, the finest, one pound. Let it stand Stirring it every day for a fortnight and then put in the honey and Treacle and two or three day after that the sugar.

Vinegar

Ingredients:

1 gallon of water
1lb of coarse [muscovado] sugar
Brown bread toast dipped in yeast

Barrel

Method: Take Gallon of water. Put a pd of the Corsest Sugar you can get and boyl 'em together. Scum it & when it is almost Cold put in a Brown Bread Tost dipt in yeast. Put it in to your Barill. So bung it up. Let it stand very warm.

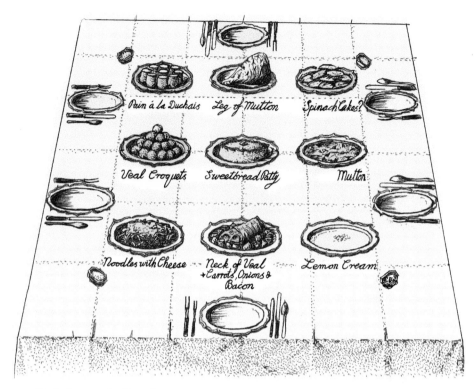

Pain à la Duchais   Leg of Mutton   Spinach Cakes?

Veal Croquets   Sweetbread Patty   Mutton

Noodles with Cheese   Neck of Veal
+ Carrots, Onions &
Bacon   Lemon Cream

19. A drawing by Peter Brears based on a plan for a dinner created by Sabine Winn. The handwritten plan itself can be found in the Nostell Priory archive at Wakefield (reference: WYW1352/4/8/6/1). Eighteenth-century dinners had a symmetrical arrangement of dishes all placed on the table at the same time, from which guests were served mainly by their hosts, but might also serve each other. Here one of Sabine's plans shows her selection of both savoury and sweet dishes for a relatively small-scale dinner.

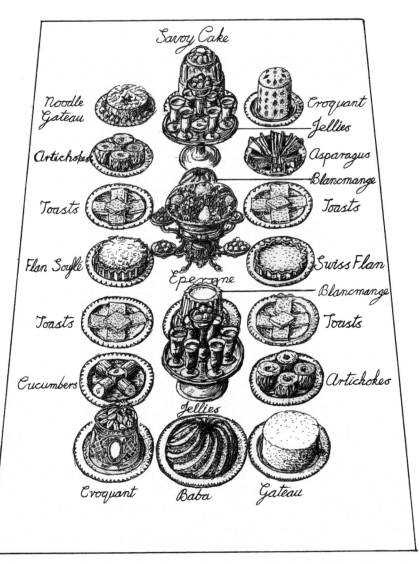

Savoy Cake

Noodle Gateau

Croquant

Jellies

Artichokes

Asparagus

Blancmange

Toasts

Toasts

Flan Soufle

Swiss Flan

Epergne

Blancmange

Toasts

Toasts

Cucumbers

Artichokes

Jellies

Croquant

Baba

Gateau

20. A drawing by Peter Brears based on another plan made by Sabine Winn, this one for the second course of a dinner for twenty people. The original handwritten plan can be found in the above-mentioned archive (reference: WYW1352/4/8/9). Twenty dishes are arranged around a central epergne. It demonstrates great skill in its arrangement, with similar dishes maintaining a diagonal symmetry, as with the croquants, hollow pierced domes of sweet pastry that usually concealed preserved fruits or ice cream.

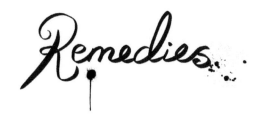

Remedies

Abdomen, Digestion and Purgatives
Admirable Beverage for Weaknesses of Constitution
Admiral Gascoigne's Tincture of Rhubarb
The Bitter Tincture
To Cause an Easy Labour
For the Colic or Gravel by Mr Cholmley
A Cordial Tincture to Treat Distempers of the Stomach, Worms,
    Gripings and Infections
Dr Macbride's Simple Remedy for the Stone
Dr Stoughton's Celebrated Stomachic Elixir
Drops for Stomach Pains
Excellent Bitter for the Stomach
Excellent Lozenges for the Heartburn
Excellent Remedy for Swelled Legs and a Relaxed Stomach
Genuine Lozenges for the Piles, as used in the West Indies
Ginger Drops
Greek Remedy for a Weak Stomach
For a Green Sickness
King Charles II's Surfeit Water
Medicine for Colic
Mrs Aylott's Excellent Remedy for Colic
A Purge for Children
A Purge for Everyone
A Purge for Head
A Purge for Poor People
Purge for Everyone Else
Red Water for Labour

Rice Jelly to Treat Weak or Infirm Constitutions
Sir Robert Ford's Drink to Sweeten the Blood
Stop a Violent Retching to Vomit
Syrup of Steel 'to prevent miscarriage'
To Treat Costiveness

Coughs, Colds and Respiratory Ailments
Agreeable Preventative of a Consumption
Aunt Barrington's Cure for Pleurisy
Cure a Cough
Cure a Horse of a Great Cold
Cure for Violent Colds and Fevers
Dr Lowther's Receipt for a Cold
Excellent Medicine for Shortness of Breath
Excellent Remedy for an Asthma
Fine Raisin Marmalade for a Cough or Cold
Galloping Consumption
Linseed Cough Syrup
Liqourice Juice
Medicine for Distemper
Pleasant Emulsion for a Cough, Cold or Hoarseness
Prevent Consumption
Rhubarb Prunes for Consumption in Children
Sage Wine, Good for a Cold Stomach
To Treat Shortness of Breath

Diseases and Disorders
For an Ague or Fever
Approved Medicine to Drive the Scurvy or any other Ill Humour out
    of a Man's Body
Broth for a Fever
Cure Convulsion Fits in those that have had Nine in a Day
Cure Fits
A Cure for all sorts of Agues
To Cure a Dropsy
Cure Madness in Dogs, Cattle etc.
Cure for Rickets

Dr Carmichael Smith's Celebrated Remedy for Preventing the Contagion
of Infectious Diseases, in Hospitals, Prisons, etc

Epileptic Electuary for the Cure of Falling Fits, Hysterics and even St
Vitus' Dance

Excellent Decoction for a Decline

Excellent Diet Drink for the Scurvy

Excellent Pills for Jaundice

An Excellent Receipt for a Violent Fever

Lurking Fever by Dr Hulse

Make Jelly of Grapes Very Good for One in a Fever

A Most Excellent Guard Against the Plague

A Most Excellent Medicine against the Plague, Smallpox, Measles,
Surfeits or Fever

Mrs Browning's Cure for Gout

Mrs Cundall's Best Cure in the World for a Dropsy

Mrs Milborn's Cure for Scabies

Mrs Milborn's Ointment for the Small Pox

Peony Powder for Fits

A Pleasant Cooling Water to Drink in a Fever

Preservative against the Plague

To Provoke Urine

For the Rheumatism, Gout & Dropsy by Mrs North

Sage Pye for Dropsy

For St Anthony's Fire

For Stoppage in the Water

To Treat Worms

For Wind in the Veins or Elsewhere

Eyes, Ears, Mouth and Skin

Aunt Dawg's Wash for the Teeth

Cure a Canker or Sore Mouth

Dr Colebatch's Remedy for Deafness

Elder Balsam

For the Eyes

Foxglove Juice for Deafness

A Hand Wash

An Incomporable Cure of the Scurvy in the Mouth

Lady Boothby's Excellent Water for the Eyes
To Make Lip Salve
To Make Pomatum
Mrs Hunter's Egg Salve for Boils
Mrs Wroth's Cure for Growths on the Eyes
Opiate for the Teeth
For a Pain in the Ear
Pommade Divine
Remedy for Deafness
Salve for Boils
Sir Thomas Haggerston's Cure for Toothache
Stinking Breath, For a
A Syrup to Kill a Canker in the Mouth
Water for the Eyes

Mental and Emotional Troubles
The Best Thing in the World for Languishing Spirits or Fatigue after a
    Journey
To Cure a Mad Dog
Dr George Cheyne's Cordial for Low Spirits, Fainting, Oppressions,
    Stomach
Sickness, Headaches and Vapours
Dr Radcliffe's Famous Diet Drink for Sharp Humours
For Vapours or any Sudden Surprise
German Method of Preventing Hysterics
To Make an Excellent Smelling Bottle
Mustard Whey for a Palsy and Nervous Disorders
Powder for Vapours Occasioned by Wind
Russian Remedy for a Vertigo

Wounds, Aches and Sores
Admirable Ointment for Burns, Scalds, Cuts, Bruises, etc.
Cephalic Snuff
To Cure a Bruise in the Eye
Cure for a Strain in the Back
Cure for Sciatica, Dropsy and Rheumatism Evil
To Cure the Sting of a Wasp or Bee

A Diet Drink to Cure all Manner of Hurts and Wounds
How to Draw a Thorn or Splinter out of Any Part of the Body
An Excellent Plaster for a Rupture
Famous American Receipt for Rheumatism
For a Headache
To Heal any Cut
Infallable Remedy for Stopping the Bleeding of the Nose
M. Homassel's Account of his Cure for Burns or Scalds
Make a Green Ointment called None Such
To Make an Eau de Luce and its use
To Make Balsamic and Anti-Putrid Vinegar for Treating Wounds
To Make the Leaden Plaster Given by Lady Dering
Oil of Brown Paper for Burns
For a Sore Breast
Speedy Cure for a Sprain
For a Violent Bleeding out of the Nose by Dr Fuller
Wash and Fomentation for an Old Wound

In his essay *A Swiss Milady in Yorkshire: Sabine Winn of Nostell Priory* (*Yorkshire Archaeological Journal*, volume 77, 2005), Professor Christopher Todd explains that Sabine's husband, Sir Rowland Winn, 5th Baronet of Nostell, suffered from consistent ill-health. In his younger years he was troubled by 'long-lasting violent headaches that had plaqued him as a teenager' and early in his marriage, on a trip to Sabine's native Switzerland, Todd describes how he'd been prone to fits of giddiness. In 1763, the couple resorted to taking in waters at Tunbridge Wells, and Todd explains that the following decade, Sir Rowland suffered from 'violent bilious attacks' along with 'gout in his right hand'.

Todd also notes Sabine Winn's reluctance to engage the services of British doctors, whom he says neither she nor her mother trusted. Indeed, ill-health was a dangerous affair in the late eighteenth century, especially with the emergence of so many quack doctors. Of course, Sabine Winn herself was partial to the supposed conjuring skills of Dr Katterfelto, who was shown up to be a fraud in later years, so it was perhaps a wise step step to compile a collection of home remedies for common complaints of the day rather than fall on the mercy of charlatans.

Late eighteenth and early nineteenth-century newspapers were full of stories about quacks poisoning their patients, featuring horrendous reports under headlines such as *DEATH BY POISONOUS MEDCINES* or *Poisoning by a Quack*. These two examples are from the 1820s, the first concerning a journeyman shoemaker from Leeds called Joseph Braithwaite, who feeling unwell had sought the advice of a Mr Charles Middleton. *The Public Ledger and Daily Advertiser* of 3 December 1827 reported how he had told a friend that he was suffering from a disease 'which required the operation of powerful medicines'. Exactly what medicines Middleton had given him, he did not know, but he told the friend that since taking them, 'he had lost the use of his arms and legs, and was compelled to creep to and from bed … and he believed it would carry him to his grave'. Undeterred, he then sought the help of another quack doctor named George Geldart of Woodhouse in Leeds. Geldart's solution was to put the patient in a warm bath. Mr Braithwaite died soon afterwards.

At the inquest, Mr Middleton said he'd been operating as a surgeon for the last six months, though he admitted he was not a member of the Royal College of Suregons. He told the coroner that he'd dispensed two pills to Mr Braithwaite: 'One of them was compounded of calomel and other ingredients, and the other of rhubarb and other ingredients.' Middleton couldn't recall exactly what quantity of each ingredient was in each pill but he boasted that he had 'some experience in the medical line' having treated thousands of patients, though what his rate of success stood at was not revealed. He recalled that one of his favoured rhubarb pills contained opium and cantharides (a poision made from Spanish fly beetles), though he didn't remember if this was what he gave the unfortunate Mr Braithwaite. He was quite sure though that whatever he gave Mr Braithwaite would not have dipossesed him of the power of his limbs. So confident was Mr Middleton of the efficacy of his drugs, he even offered to take double the dosage given to Mr Braithwaite before the assembled jury to prove their lack of poisoness contents. The offer was declined.

An expert witness in the form of Mr Hay, a Leeds surgeon, examined the body, noting inflammation of the stomach and bowels, and concluded that the deceased had died as a direct result of taking too large a dose of the drugs administered by Mr Middleton. The jury returned the following verdict: 'That the deceased died of inflammation of the stomach and bowels, occasioned by incautiously taking and swallowing poison in too large quantities, when using it as medicine.'

The second headline cited above referred to an incident that took place in Edinburgh a year earlier and was reported in the *Berkshire Chronicle* on 12 August 1826. A Dr Campbell had visited a spirit merchant's shop to purchase whisky and noted that the young shop assistant had a 'small stoppage in one of his nostrils'. The self-styled doctor offered to remove it for him in exchange for a small sum. Agreeing to the terms, the young man drank a liquid from a vial that the doctor had taken from his coat pocket. Immediately the patient fell ill. He was 'seized with a sickness and violent gripiness about the stomach' and was soon unable to remain on his feet. A local GP was called and he administered a purgative, which undid the damage.

It was later revealed that Dr Campbell's remedy had consisted of a 'considerable quantity of the solution of corrosive sublimate (a powerful poison)'. Campbell was arrested. In his defence he claimed that the remedy had worked on many hundreds of previous patients and if he was allowed to walk free from custody he would sign a piece of paper vowing to leave the town forever!

Most of Sabine Winn's receipts, and those published by our unnamed friend in 1807 and 1815, are of a more homeopathic nature, but several contain substances that would be quite dangerous to handle or consume.

Each remedy is organised into one of six catergories. The first covers abdominal and digestive complaints such as heartburn, piles, colic and weak stomachs, purgatives or purges being popular remedies. One of these purges is made with sherry. It is followed by an almost exact version but this time sherry is substituted for water and this is genuinely described in the original receipt book as a 'purge for poor people'.

Then there are cures for coughs, colds and respiratory ailments, the common cold being a real menace then as now, evidenced by the sheer number of cold remedies found in the original source material. Contemporary diseases such as consumption (usually pulmonary tuberculosis) carried off many unfortunate sufferers in this era. And during the nineteenth century, phthisis (another term for consumption) was a common cause of death noted on many death certificates issued from 1837, so it's unsurprising that the receipt books contain several supposed remedies for this complaint, with one rather tragically titled *Rhubarb Prunes for Consumption in Children*. Another cure for a cold comes in the form of *Liquorice Juice*. From the sixteenth century, liquorice had a good reputation for warding off coughs and colds. The main source of English liquorice was Pontefract, only 4½ miles from Nostell, where the bushes were grown and their roots dug up for processing. It is interesting to follow Sabine's recipe for extracting juice from the roots, first mixing it with gum and sugar, then forming it into rolls before drying them in the form of short, thin black sticks. This method was first published in 'W. M.'s' *A Queen's Delight* in 1655.

Next come remedies for diseases and disorders. This is a wide-ranging selection, including a cure for the disease rickets, which caused children's bones to weaken or soften usually owing to a lack vitamin D or minerals in the diet. Another contemporary disease was known as dropsy, where fluid builds up under the skin, today known as edema or oedema. Whether 1 quart of white wine, ¼lb of Castile soap and 1 spoonful of olive oil actually removed the symptoms is unclear but it was claimed that this receipt was the *'Best Cure in the World for Dropsy'*.

Problems of the eyes, ears, mouth and skin follow and there's a remedy for toothache, along with a receipt for a form of toothpaste called *Aunt Dawg's Wash for the Teeth*. There's also a receipt for a hand wash that was made from almonds, raisins, ox gall, fortified wine and 2 or 3 eggs. Ox gall is used today as part of a wetting agent in engraving and watercolour painting. There are remedies for deafness, eye washes, a version of *Pommade Divine* for the skin, and for those with bad, or *Stinking Breath*, a receipt made from just boiled coriander seeds and fortified wine.

Then come receipts for mental and emotional troubles, and three are different cures for fits of the vapours – an archaic disease supposed to cause fainting and low moods, which was attributed to women and so called because it was thought that vapours from the womb were responsible. This section also includes a Russian remedy for vertigo and a German method for preventing hysterics.

The last selection, covering wounds, aches and sores, contains probably the most useful receipts for use on a day to day basis, offering remedies for such misfortunes as bee or wasp stings, back strains, headaches, cuts and bruises, burns and even a method for withdrawing a splinter 'out of any part of the body'.

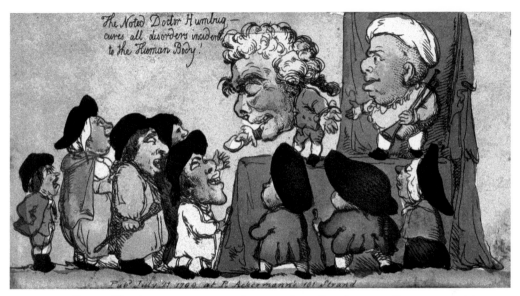

21. Doctor Humbug, an itinerant medicine vendor selling his wares from a stage with the aid of an assistant, 1799.

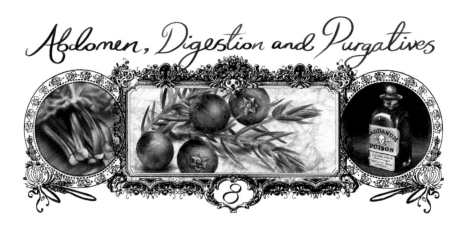

Admirable Beverage for Weaknesses of Constitution
(1807)

Ingredients:

Pearl barley
1oz gum Arabic

Method: The most distressing weaknesses, with which delicate constitutions are so often afflicted, may be better cured by simply substituting the following beverage for the usual drink of beer, ale, &c. at meal times, during a few days or weeks, according to the degree of weakness, than the most costly and complicated medicines. Boil as much pearl or Scotch barley, in pure water, as will make about three pints; then, straining it off, and having in the meantime dissolved an ounce of gum Arabic in a little water, mix them, and just boil the whole up together. The barley water need not be thick, as the gum will give it sufficient consistence. When used, take it milk warm; the good effect will generally be soon manifest, and a compleat cure certainly follow.

Admiral Gascoigne's Tincture of Rhubarb
(1807)

Ingredients:

½oz of powdered rhubarb
½oz of powdered myrrh
½oz of cochineal
½oz of hiera picra
2 pints of double-distilled aniseed water

Method: Take half an ounce each of powdered rhubarb, myrrh, cochineal, anti hiera-picra, and put them in a bottle with one quart of the best double-distilled aniseed water: When it has stood four days, it is fit for immediate use; and may be taken, a small wine-glassful at a time, for any pains in the stomach or bowels. In the valuable old manuscript collection from which this is extracted, is the following memorandum – 'There is not a better receipt in the world!'

The Bitter Tincture

Ingredients:

1 dram of saffron
1 dram of salt of wormwood
2 drams of sliced gentian root
2 drams of Virginia Snakeroot, cut small
2 drams of dried orange peal
2 drams of chamomile flowers
½ dram of cochineal in fine powder

Method: Put the ingredients into a glass bottle & pour on 'em an English pint of good French Brandy. Cork the bottle & let it stand near the fire or in the sun for 5 or 6 days. Shake the bottle once or twice a day & when fine decant it. Take 40 drops morning & afternoon in a glass of strong white wine.

To Cause an Easy Labour

Ingredients:

6oz of brown sugar candy, beaten into powder
¼lb of raisins of the sun (stoned)
2oz of dates (unstoned and sliced)
1oz of aniseeds (bruised)
¼oz of cowslip flowers
A dram of rosemary flowers
4 pints of white wine

A flint stone
A porous bag

Method: Gather together the listed ingredients ten or twelve days before her looking [ready to give birth]. Put these into a fine lawn bag with a flint stone (that it may sink) into the white wine. Let it steep 24 hours and after take of it in the morning, at four in the afternoon and in the evening. The quantity is a wine glass full.

For the Colic or Gravel by Mr Cholmley

Ingredients:

3oz of Senna
2oz of elecampane roots, aniseed, coriander seeds, guaiacum
3 x 3 quarts and a pint of brandy

Method: Take of the best Senna three ounces, elicompany roots, Anniseeds, Coriander seeds, Guiacum, of each two ounces. Put to these three 3 quarts and a Pint of Brandy. Let them infuse four days, stir them once or twice a day, then strain them thro' a Flannel for use. The dose is three or four spoonsful.

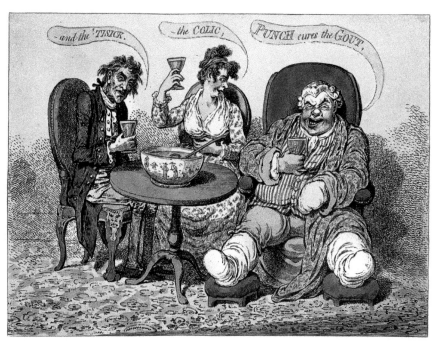

22. An obsese gouty man drinking punch. By J. Gillray in 1799 and published by H. Humphrey in *Catalogue of Political and Personal Satires.*

A Cordial Tincture to Treat Distempers of the Stomach, Worms, Gripings and Infections

Ingredients:

1 handful of:
   Angelica
   Cardus Benedictus
   Juniper berries
2 handfuls of wormwood
Spirits of wine
White wine, for serving

Wide-mouth bottle

Method: Take of Angelico, Cardus Benedictus & Juniper berries a handful of Each and of Wormwood 2 handfulls. Pick these and Dry them and put them into a wide mouth bottle then pour on them as m'ch spiritt of Wine as will cover them an Inch high. Let this stand 14 dayes after pour it off and Keepe it for your use as you want it. Power into a Draught of White Wine 10 or 12 drops of the aforesaid Tincture or if Occasion be 20. It is good in all Distempers of the Stomack, good against wormes and all gripeings and admirable against all infection. It can not be Given amise.

Dr Macbride's Simple Remedy for the Stone
(1807)

Ingredients:

30 unroasted coffee berries, otherwise coffee cheeries
10 drops of spirit of nitre
1 or 2 spoonsful of castor oil

Method: Boil thirty unroasted coffee-berries in a quart of water, till the liquid becomes of a greenish hue; half a pint of which is to be taken every morning and evening, with ten drops of the sweet spirit of nitre. It will be proper, while using this medicine, occasionally to open the bowels by taking a spoonful or two of castor oil. This simple remedy is said to have been administered with great success, in this most painful and dangerous disease.

Dr Stoughton's Celebrated Stomachic Elixir
(1807)

Ingredients:

The rinds of 6 large Seville oranges
1oz gentian root, scraped and sliced
½ dram of cochineal
1 pint of brandy

Method: Pare off the thin yellow rinds of six large Seville oranges and put them in a quart bottle, with an ounce of gentian root scraped and sliced, and half a dram of cochineal. Pour over these ingredients a pint of the best brandy; shake the bottle well, several times, during that and the following day; let it stand two days more to settle; and clear it off into bottles for use. Take one or two tea-spoonfuls, morning and afternoon, in a glass of wine, or even in a cup of tea. This is an elegant but simple preparation, little differing from the compound tincture of gentian either of the London or Edinburgh Dispensatories; the former adding half an ounce of canella alba; and the latter only substituting for the cochineal of Stoughton, half an ounce of husked and bruised seeds of the lesser cardamom. In deciding on their respective merits, it should seem, that Stoughton's elixir has the advantage in simplicity; and, perhaps, altogether, as a general and elegant stomachic. Indeed, for some- particular intentions, both the London and Edinburgh compositions may have their respective claims to preference: in a cold stomach, the cardamom might be useful, and, in a laxative habit, the canella alba. As a family medicine, however, to be at all times safely resorted to, we need not hesitate to recommend Dr Stoughton's elixir.

Drops for Stomach Pains

Ingredients:

2 pints of brandy
1oz of gentian root, cut into pieces
½oz of saffron
Peel of 9 Seville oranges
White wine, for serving
Cochineal (optional)

Method: A quart of brandy, an ounce of Gentian, cut into peices, half an ounce of Saffron, the peel of 9 sevel Orinces steep'd & shaken 8 or 9 days, then draw it off & take a bout a Tea spoonfull in a glass of w't wine. You may add a little cocheneal.

Excellent Bitter for the Stomach
(1815)

Ingredients:

1oz gentian root, sliced
1oz fresh rind of lemon
2 drachms of cardamom seeds, bruised
3 drachms of Seville orange peel
1½ pints of boiling water

Method: Take one ounce of gentian root sliced, one ounce of fresh rind of lemon, two drachms of cardamom seeds bruised, three drachms of Seville orange peel; pour a pint and a half of boiling water over the ingredients, let it stand an hour, then decant the clear liquor, and take a wine glass full two or three times a day. It should be kept closely covered after the water is put in the ingredients.

Excellent Lozenges for the Heartburn
(1807)

Ingredients:

Calcined oyster shells
½lb sugar
1 spoonful of milk
1 spoonful of water

Method: Take calcined oyster-shells; as found on the sea-coast, where they are so blanched by time as to appear, both within and without, of the whiteness of mother of pearl, dry them well by the fire, and then beat and sift them as fine as possible. In half a pound of this powder, mix half a pound of loaf sugar well beaten and sifted; and wet it with a spoonful or two of milk and water, so as to form a very stiff paste. Then mould the whole into neat lozenges, of any form or size, and bake them very dry in so slack an oven as not to discolour them; this will be best effected, after every' thing else is drawn. These lozenges so effectually destroy that acidity in the stomach which causes this complaint, as not only to prevent the disagreeable sensation it occasions, but greatly to promote digestion. Their power in neutralizing acids may be easily tried, by dissolving one of them in a glass of the sharpest vinegar.

Excellent Remedy for Swelled Legs and a Relaxed Stomach
(1807)

Ingredients:

6oz of common bitter infusion:
    Gentian root
    Outer rind of Seville orange
    Coriander seeds, optional
    1oz tincture of senna
    1 dram of compound of spirts of lavender
Marshmallow leaves
Rue
Chamomile
Southernwood
2 pints of ale

Method: Take six ounces of the common bitter infusion, consisting of gentian root and outer rind of Seville orange, with or without coriander seeds; one ounce of tincture of senna; and a dram of compound spirits of lavender. Mix them together, and take four spoonfuls every other night on going to bed. To prevent swelled legs from breaking, make a decoction of marsh-mallow leaves, rue, camomile, and southern wood, boiled in a quart of ale or stale beer, and foment them with flannels wrung out of the liquor, as hot as can be borne without scalding, three or four times a day. After bathing, anoint them with a little ointment of marsh-mallows; and, should they even be broke, only cover the holes with dry lint, while bathing or fomenting the legs, and afterwards dress them with the ointment, and take a little cooling physic.

Genuine Lozenges for the Piles, as used in the West Indies
(1807)

Ingredients:

4oz powdered sugar
2oz of flour of sulpher
Gum tacamahaca
Rose water

Method: Take four ounces of fine powdered loaf sugar, two ounces of flour of sulphur, and a sufficient quantity of mucilage of gum tacamahaca dissolved in red rose water to form the whole into a paste for lozenges. Having made it up in lozenges of the desired form, dry them before the fire, or in an oven after every thing has been drawn. Take, of these lozenges, about the weight of a dram daily. This is a most valuable medicine for that disagreeable and dreadful complaint; which prevails much, and is a peculiarly grievous and even dangerous disease in the West India Islands, as well as in most other hot climates. It is, however, generally found compleatly efficacious, even there.

Ginger Drops
(1807)

Ingredients:

1oz of candied orange peel
½lb sugar
½oz powdered ginger

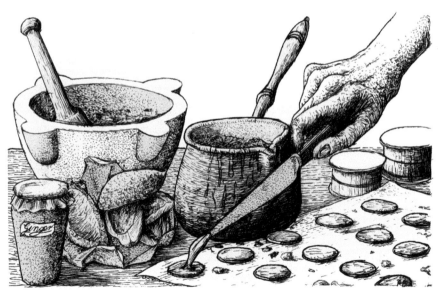

23. Ginger drops by Peter Brears. Ginger drops were made of ground ginger, pulverised candied peel and sugar boiled together to form a thick syrup. Having been dropped onto a sheet of paper from the tip of a knife, they set hard before being stored in boxes, ready to cure colds.

Method: These drops, which are excellent for a cold stomach, may be made in the following easy manner: Beat, in a marble mortar, an ounce of the best candied orange peel, with a little loaf sugar; and, when it becomes a smooth paste, add half a pound of loaf sugar, and half an ounce of the best powdered ginger. Then, with a little water to dissolve the sugar, boil the whole to a candy, or carimel, and drop it off from the point of a knife on writing paper, in small round drops, about the size of a silver two-pence. When quite cold, they will come off the paper, and are to be kept in papered boxes. Among other good qualities of ginger, it is said to be beneficial in dimness of sight &c.

Greek Remedy for a Weak Stomach
(1807)

Ingredients:

1 pint of wine
1 dram of powdered myrrh or frankincense, wormwood and
  castor

Method: Infuse, in a pint of wine, one dram each of powdered myrrh, thus or frankincense, wormwood, and castor, for eight or ten days; of which, take a glass after dinner, and it will excellently assist digestion.

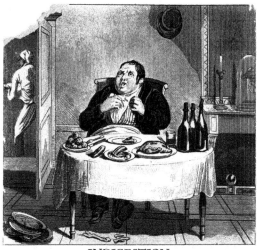

INDIGESTION

24. A corpulent gentleman with indigestion. Line engraving, c. eighteenth century.

For a Green Sickness

Ingredients:

A dram of the best rhubarb
½oz of Aloes
1oz of rusty steel filings
A little white wine
A little liquorice powder

Method: First take a vomit. Take the Dram of the best Rubarb in powd'r, Half an Oun: of Aloes, an Oun: of rusty Steel Fileings. Wet 'em with a little white wine & roll 'em in a little Liquorish powder. This quantity will make near a 100 pills whereof take 2 at night & 3 in the morning washing 'em down with a little warm Ale. Keep your neck & hands warm & do not dabble in Cold Water. Take 'em 2 dayes & rest one 'till you have taken 40 pills.

King Charles the Second's Surfeit Water
(1807)

Ingredients:

1 gallon of fine brandy
2 pints of aniseed cordial water
1lb fine sugar
1 pint of poppy water
1 pint of rose water
1½lb stoned jar raisins
¼lb new dates, stoned and sliced
1oz bruised cinnamon and cloves
4 pounded nutmegs
1 stick of scraped and sliced liquorice

Method: The surfeit waters were formerly much in vogue, and the modes of preparation very numerous, but they are now scarcely known in medicine. We should, at least, preserve one of them in this collection; and, undoubtedly, this is one of the best. Pour a gallon of the finest brandy, a quart of aniseed cordial water, and a pint each of poppy and red rose waters, into a large stone bottle; on a pound of fine powdered sugar, a pound and a half of stoned jar raisins, a quarter of a pound of fine new dates stoned and sliced; an ounce each of bruised cinnamon and cloves, four pounded nutmegs, and a stick of scraped and sliced liquorice. Let the whole infuse nine days closely stopped, and well stirred or shook four times daily. Then add three pounds of fresh red poppy flowers, or three large handfuls of dried flowers; with a sprig of angelica, and two or three sprigs of balm: and, when it has stood a week longer, being stirred or shook daily in like manner, strain it off, and bottle it for use.

Medicine for Colic

Ingredients:

½oz of asafoetida
1 dram of saffron, powdered
½ pint of pennyroyal water
½ pint of compound peony water
½ pint of rue water
½oz of tincture of castor

Method: Take assa-Fatida half an Ounce, Saffron in powder: one Dram. Put them in a morter and pour upon 'em by Degrees the following things, and besure they be well mixed. Penny Royal water, Compound Peony water, Rue water, each half a pint, Tincture of Caster half an ounce. You must take 4 or 5 spoounfulls of this when you find the fit comeing upon you, but be sure to shake the Bottle well first. Take of the same quantity whenever your spirits are low or if you have any other Disorder upon you, eather night or day.

Mrs Aylott's Excellent Remedy for Colic

Ingredients:

1oz of the best rhubarb
2 pints of sack, otherwise fortified wine

Method: Slice an Ounce of the best Rubarb into a quart of Sack 12 hours. Then drink 4 spoonfulls once a day for 6 or 8 weeks together. Fill up your Bottle as you empty it. When the virtue of the Rubarb is spent, put in fresh. It must be constantly continued 'till the Bowells & Blood are strengthened.

A Purge for Children

Ingredients:

¼oz of rhubarb
½oz of Senna
½oz of liquorice
¼oz of aniseed
1 pint of ale
A few stoned raisins

Method: Slice the Rhub: & Liquorish & bruise the seeds. Put all into a pint of Ale with a few raisons ston'd. Let it infuse 'till 'tis strong of the things, then give in the morning 2 or 3 spoonfulls, more or less, as you find it work. If it works but 3 times in a day, repeat it 3 or 4 days together. You may put in a little creame of tartar if you please.

A Purge for Everyone

Ingredients:

Peach leaves or blossoms
Warm water
Sugar

Method: Take peache leaves or blossoms enfused in warm water for 24 houers. Then strane it out and put new in as before and renewe it 6 times. Then strane the licker and boyle up with suger to a syrop. Take 2 sponfulls at a time.

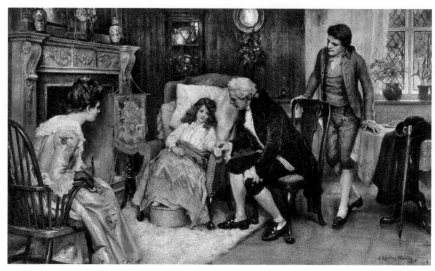

25. A Georgian physician is attending a sick girl; father in the background, mother seated in an armchair in the foreground. Photogravure after G.S. Knowles, 1906.

A Purge for the Head

Ingredients:

1oz of Senna
½oz of rhubarb
½oz of sweet fennel seeds
1 quart of strong white wine

Method: Cut the rhubarb thin, bruise the seeds, steep 'em 24 hours in a quart of strong white wine. Take it 3 mornings together a 3rd part of it at a time. If it works oftener than 3 times in a day, then take it each other day.

A Purge for Poor People...

Ingredients:

1oz of hiera picra
1 pint of aniseed water

Method: Take 1 Oun: of Hyra Picra and put into it a pint of Anniseed water. Let it stand 4 or 5 days shaking it often. Pour off the clear. Take of it 3 spoonfulls goeing to bed & 3 in the morning. Before you take this Purge take a gentle Vomit.

… And one for Everyone Else

Ingredients:

2oz of hiera picra
2 pints of sherry

Method: Take 2 ounces of Hyra Piera. Put it into a quart bottle of Sherry. Let it stand 4 or 5 days, shakeing it often. Pour off the clear. Take 3 spoonfulls of it going to bed & 3 in the morning. Before you take this purge, take a gentle vomit.

Red Water for Labour
(1807)

Ingredients:

3 pints of brandy
1 dram of hiera picra
4 drams of liquorice powder
1 dram of cochineal
1lb sugar candy

Method: Put three pints of brandy, one dram of hiera picra, four drams of liquorice powder, and a dram of cochineal, in a bottle; and, setting it by the fire side for eight days, often shaking it, strain it through a flannel bag, and put to it a pound of sugar candy. This is highly recommended to procure labour and afterpains, bring away a false conception, &c.

Rice Jelly to Treat Weak or Infirm Constitutions
(1807)

Ingredients:

¼lb of rice flour
½lb sugar
2 pints of water

Method: This is one of the best and most nourishing preparations of rice, particularly for valetudinarians. It is thus made. Boil a quarter of a pound of rice flour, with half a pound of loaf sugar, in a quart of water, till the whole becomes one uniform gelatinous mass; then strain off the jelly, and let it stand to cool. If, of this light, nutritious, and salubrious food, a little be frequently eaten, it will be found very beneficial to all weakly and infirm constitutions.

Sir Robert Ford's Drink to Sweeten the Blood

Ingredients:

1½ drams of:
  Sarsaparilla
  Roasted China, sliced thin
1 pint of boiling water
15–20 Guernsey sage leaves
Sugar, to sweeten
15–20 grains of senna (optional)
Manna, to sweeten (optional)

Method: Take of Sarsparilla one drahm & halfe a China rosted the Like quantity sliced thin. Put it into your tea pot, pour upon it a pint of Water boiling hot. Let it infuse a quarter of an houre close stoped then add 15 or 20 leaves of gernsy sage & within a quarter of an oure poure it out & sweeten it to your tast. To be Drunk after diner & at night. If you would have it Purging add to your morning Infusion 15 or 20 graines of Sena & in stede of Sugar Sweeten it with manna.

Stop a Violent Retching to Vomit

Ingredients:

1 tea spoonful of lemon juice
1 tea spoonful of spirit of lavender
30 drops of liquid laudanum

Method: Mix all together in a spoon and give it to the patient. It will stay the retching, give ease and compose to sleep.

Syrup of Steel, 'to prevent miscarriage'

Ingredients:

1oz of steel filings
1 pint of white wine
½ dram of mace
Sugar, enough to create a thin syrup

Paper suitable for straining
Bottle

Method: Take 1 ounce of Filings of Steel. Put into it a Pint of White Wine. Let it stand 3 weeks then Pour it off into another bottle. Put in half a Dram of Mace, bruised. Let it stand a week to infuse then Pour it off through Cap Paper into a bottle and then Desolve as much Loaf Suger broken but not Powdered as will make it into a thin Surrap with out boyling. Take every morning a Spoonfull for 3 or 4 Months together. This is good to prevent miscaring.

To Treat Costiveness

Ingredients:

¼lb of virgin honey
Cream of tartar
Gruel, made with water
Common mallows
Butter

Method: Take Virgin Honey a quart'r of a pound & mix it with as much Cream of Tarter as will bring it to a pritty thick Electuary, of which take the bigness of a Walnut when you please & for your Breakfast eat Water-gruel with Common mallows boiled in it & a good piece of butter, the mallows must be chopt small & eaten with the Gruel.

9

Agreeable Preventative of a Consumption
(1807)

Ingredients:

2 new-laid eggs
Rose water
Powdered cinnamon
Sugar

Method: Set two new-laid eggs in hot embers, till they are thoroughly warm, but without suffering the whites to get hard; then make, a small hole on the top of each egg, pour off the whites as expeditiously as possible. and fill up the eggs with red-rose water, and powdered cinnamon and sugar; warm them again in the embers; and eat them as soon as they are sufficiently done, This constantly repeated, at least once every day, will generally prove very effectual in preventing a decline.

Aunt Barrington's Cure for Pleurisy

Ingredients:

Greenest broom
Ale, enough to cover the broom
Mithridate, the size of a hazelnut

4-pint skillet

Method: Fill a 2 quart Skillet w'th the Greenest Broom you can get. Cut an Inch Long almost to the top then put in ale, enough to cover it, & let it boyle to 12 Spoonfulls. Strain it out, then take 4 spoonfulls of it & put the bignesse of Hasell nut of Methridate to it & take it at night goeing to bed. Do so for 3 nights together.

Cure a Cough

Ingredients:

Garlic
Spring water
Sugar
Egg whites

Method: Take of garlick a good quantity, pick it & slice them small then boile them in spring water very well 'till halfe be consumed. Do so 3 or 4 times untill the garlick hath lost some what of its tast & smell. To the last Liquor add its full Proportion of Sugar. Clarifie it w'th the whites of Eggs & boile to the consistence of a sirup. When tis cold bottle it up for use. Probatum est.

Cure a Horse of a Great Cold

Ingredients:

2 pints of ale
½lb of treacle
1 garlic head
Warm water

Method: Take a Quart of Ale, Half a p'd of Treacle & a head of Garlick. Give it Him 3 Moarnings together blood warm, fasting an hour after it, then let him drink a little warm water.

Cure for Violent Colds and Fevers
(1807)

Ingredients:

½oz of pearl barley
3 pints of water
½oz powdered spermaceti
½oz nitre drops
Honey

Method: The following remedy will prove highly beneficial to every person afflicted with a cold and fever, however violent; and seldom fails of relief, either in young or old. Boil half an ounce of pearl barley in about three pints of water, till half reduced; then add half an ounce of powdered spermaceti, with half an ounce of nitre drops, and. sweeten the whole with genuine Narbonne honey. The dose is two table-spoonfuls, to be taken thrice a day; the party, in the mean time, being carefully kept from exposure to fresh cold.

Dr Lower's Receipt for a Cold

Ingredients:

2 spoonsful of the best salad oil
¼lb of brown sugar candy, finely beaten with the juice of half a lemon

Method: Mix these together and take of it at your pleasure.

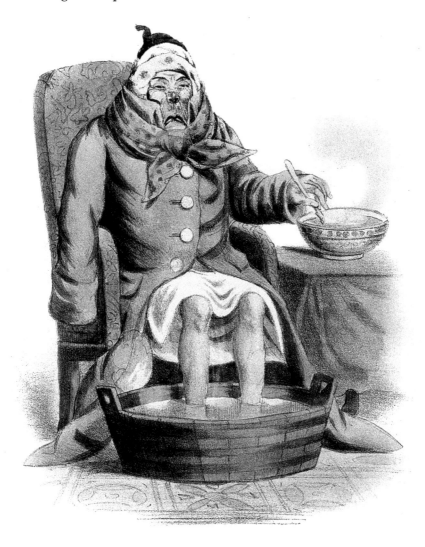

Excellent Medicine for Shortness of Breath
(1807)

Ingredients:

¾oz of finely powdered senna
½oz of flour of brimstone
¼oz of pounded ginger
4oz of clarified honey

Method: Mix three quarters of an ounce of finely powdered senna, half an ounce of flour of brimstone, and a quarter of an ounce of pounded ginger, and four ounces of clarified honey. Take the bigness of a nutmeg' every night and morning, for five days successively; afterwards once a week, for some time; and, finally, once a fortnight.

Excellent Remedy for an Asthma
(1807)

Ingredients:

½oz of zedoary
2 drams and ½ of flour of brimstone
1 dram of gum ammoniac
½ dram of saffron
3 pints of hydromel, or sweetened water

Method: Boil half an ounce of zedoary, two drams and a half of flour of brimstone, a dram and a half of gum ammoniac, and half a dram of saffron, in three pints of hydromel, or water sweetened at discretion with honey, till reduced to a quart. Drink an ounce of this cold, three times a day; in the morning fasting, at five in the afternoon, and on going to rest.

Fine Raisin Marmalade for a Cough or Cold
(1807)

Ingredients:

6oz of Malaga raisins
6oz of sugar candy
1oz conserve of roses
25 drops of vitriol
20 drops of oil of sulphur

Method: Stone six ounces of the best Malaga raisins, and beat them to a very fine paste with the same quantity of sugar-candy; then add an ounce of conserve of roses, twenty-five drops of oil of vitriol, and twenty drops of oil of sulphur. Mix the whole well together, and take about the quantity of a nutmeg night and morning. A smaller quantity will be sufficient for children, proportioned to their age.

Galloping Consumption

Ingredients:

½lb of raisins of the sun, stoned
¼lb of figs
¼lb of honey
½oz of *Lucatellus's* Balsam
½oz of powder of steel
½oz of flour of elecampane
1 grated nutmeg
½lb of double refined sugar, pounded

Also…

1 pint of salad oil
1 glass of old Malaga sack [fortified wine]
1 yolk of a newly laid egg
½ oz of flour of Brimstone

Method: Shred and pound all these together in a Stone-Mortar; pour into it a Pint of Sallad Oil by Degrees. Eat a Bit of it four Times a Day, the Bigness of a Nutmeg. Every Morning drink a Glass of Old *Malaga* Sack, with the Yolk of a new laid Egg, and as much Flour of Brimstone as will lie upon a Six-pence; the next Morning as much Flour of Elicampane, alternately.

Linseed Cough Syrup
(1807)

Ingredients:

1oz of linseed oil
2 pints of water
6oz moist sugar
2oz sugar candy
½oz of liquorice
Juice of 1 lemon
2 tablespoons of good rum

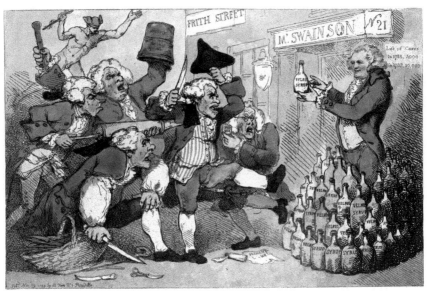

26. Isaac Swainson promoting his 'Velnos syrup'. By Thomas Rowlandson in 1789 and published by W. Fores.

Method: Boil an ounce of linseed in a quart of water, till half wasted; then add six ounces of moist sugar, two ounces of sugar candy, half an ounce of Spanish liquorice, and the juice of a large lemon. Let the whole slowly simmer together, till it becomes of a syrupy consistence; and, when cold, put to it two table-spoonfuls of the best old rum.

Liquorice Juice

Ingredients:

2lb of liquorice roots
3 gallons of spring water, plus an extra 4 or 5 spoonsful
1lb of sugar candy
A quarter of an ounce of gum

Stone mortar
3-pint skillet

Method: Take two pound of Liquourish & scrape it very clean & slice it thinne, the length of your finger, then steepe in a Gallon of spring water all night. Next day take two gallons of water more and put to it & boile it foure houres, then take it up & beate it very well in a stone morter & put it into the liquour again & boile it three houres longer. Then take it and strain it into a three pint skillit & keepe it warme. Then you must have it stirring whilst it is very thick upon a fire that will keep it warme. Then you must have one pound of sieved sugar candy. Then you must have a quarter of an ounce of gumme & steep it all night in foure or five spoonfulls of spring water. In the morning beate it but first put the water from it then put a Little sugar candy to this & the Liquourish and beate it all together upon a plate 'till it works up and so work it with sugar like to a past[e] then roll it & lay it dry but you must dry it on a paper in a stove.

Medicine for Distemper

Ingredients:

1oz of fine Peruvian bark
1 dram of castor oil
1 dram of nutmegs
½ pint of:
   Pennyroyal water
   Rue water
   Compound peony water
½oz of compound spirit of lavender
2 oz of peony syrup

12 papers

Method: Take fine Peruvain Bark one Ounce, Rupeia Castor and nutmegs of each a Dram. Make them into fine powder and divide it into 12 papers. Take penny Royall water, Rue and Compound Peony Water of each half a pint, Compound Sp'r of Lavand'r half an ounce, Syrup of Peony 2 Ounces. Mix them and make them into a Julep and upon your well Days, first in the morning and at 4 in the after noon and Last at night take one of these papers of powder and put it into a Wine Glass of the Julep at these times provided your Distemp'r Intermits. This is Counted Infallible.

Pleasant Emulsion for a Cough, Cold, or Hoarseness
(1807)

Ingredients:

½ pint of hyssop water
½oz of oil of almonds
2oz sugar

Method: Mix half a pint of hyssop water, half an ounce of oil of almonds and two ounces of powdered loaf sugar. Take a table-spoonful every night and morning. If there be any rawness or soreness of the throat or breast, add two tea-spoonsful of Friar's balsam or Turlington's drops.

To Prevent Consumption

Ingredients:

1 gallon of milk from a red cow
80 snail shells
1 handful of spearmint
White sugar candy, to sweeten

Stone mortar
Distiller
Porringer, for serving

Method: Take a Gallon of red Cows milk. Put into it 80 Snailes bruis'd Shells & all in a Stone-mortar & put in a good handfull of spearmint. Distill it off & drink a small porringer of it every morning warm'd, sweeten it with white sugar Candy.

Rhubarb Prunes, for Constipation in Children

Ingredients:

½oz of rhubarb
Nearly ½oz of senna
1lb of prunes

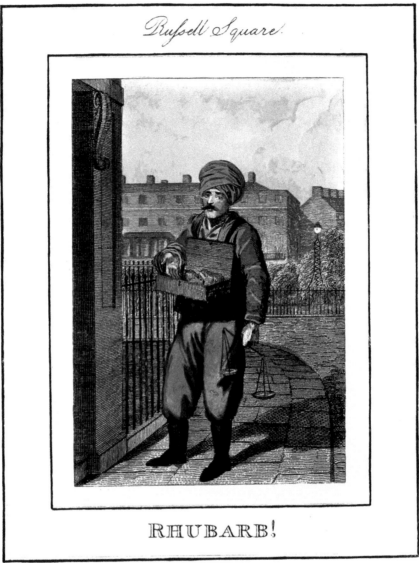

Russell Square

RHUBARB!

Craig. del.   Published April. 25.1804. by Richard Phillips. 71. S.t Pauls Church Yard.

27. A Turkish rhubarb seller from *Modern London*, 1804.

Method: Take half an ounse of rubord & near as much sena and strew them in a pound of proons and let the Chealdorn take 4 or 5 in a morning fasting, & more after if thay do not work with them.

Sage Wine, Good for a Cold Stomach

Ingredients:

½ a bushel of sage, picked from the stalks
3lb of stoned raisins
4 gallons of water
3lb of white sugar
2 pints of Canary wine

Method: Take half a bushell of red-sage pick't from the stalks, wash & dry it well, 3 pound of rasons stone'd, beat 'em well together, then put it into a stone pot, then boyle 4 Gallons of water, 'till one wastes. Then take it off from the Fire, pour it to the Sage & Rasons, cover it up close 24 hours, then strain it thro' a bag, do not squeeze it. Put 3 pd. of white sugar to it. Fan it up putting in a quart of Canary. Let it stand a Fortnight, Bottle it off.

To Treat Shortness of Breath

Ingredients:

Elecampane roots
2 handfuls of:
    Hyssop
    Pennyroyal
    Liquorice
1 gallon of pure water

Method: Let them drink a good draught of this drink every day first and last and one hour after diner for the space of 8 dayes and it will help, God willing. Take the roots of Ellecampane, cut it in small peices, of hyssop & penyroyall and good scraped Liquoras of each 2 handfull, seeth them in a Gallon of pure and fare water untill it comes to one pottle then straine it & keep it in a clean vessel close stopd and use it as afores'd.

Diseases and Disorders

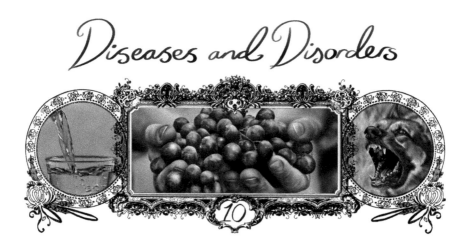

10

For an Ague or Fever

Ingredients:

3oz of Jesuit's bark, powdered
2 pints of strong white wine or sherry

Quart bottle

Method: Take 3 ounces of the best Jesuits Bark powder'd very fine. Put in a quart bottle. Fill the bottle with strong white wine or sherry, shake it well together & let it stand at least 24 hours then as soon as the fit is fully off, let Him drink a wine Glass full of the clear. Then fill the bottle up again & shake it & let Him fast an hour. Then three hours after his drinking the first glasse let him drink another glass & so every 3 hours night & day 'till the time of the next fit is fully off then take it 3 times a day until the time of 2 fits be off. Then take morning & night for a week & then 3 days before the change & full of the moon for 2 or 3 Moons. You must always fill up your Bottle still as he drinks & give it a shake each time. He must not purge after it, & he must fast an hour before he drinks as well as after.

An Approved Medicine to Drive the Scurvy or any other Ill Humour out of a Man's Body

Ingredients:

1 pint of running water
The flesh of three lemons
2 or 3 sprigs of rosemary
A quantity of sliced figs

Some raisins of the sun (stoned)
A few aniseeds (bruised)
Some sliced liquorice
Powdered white sugar candy

Method: Boyle all these together to a pint, then put in as much white sugar candy (powered) as will make it a syrup. Then let 'em boyle together and scum it. Let the party drink of it two spoonsful at a time, twice or thrice in a day.

Broth for a Fever

Ingredients:

6 pints of water
¼lb of currants
A little oatmeal
1 handful of fennel roots
1 handful of twitch grass (otherwise couch grass) roots
1 handful of suckery roots
1 small handful of parsley roots

Method: Take 3 quarts of Water, a quart'r of a pound of Currance, a little Oatmeal, a handfull of Fennell roots, a handfull of twich grass roots, Suckery-roots, a handfull, & a little handfull of Parsley roots. Boyle it enough & drink of it often.

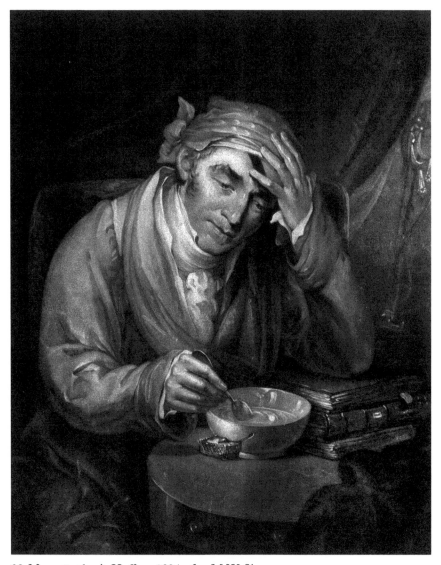

28. Mezzotint by A. Huffam, 1826, after M.W. Sharp.

Cure Convulsion Fits in those that have had Nine in a Day

Ingredients:

Equal quantities of:
  Raw onions
  Black pepper
Mithridate, or syrup of oil of amber
Black cherry water
Peony, clove and gillyflower syrup
Peony root necklace

Method: Take the ingredients stamped pretty small and lay it at the soles of the feet. Force 'em not to take anything inwardly, but anoint the wrists, the palms of the hands, the temples and the nostrils with Mithridate, amber being too hot for a child. Between the fits let 'em drink black cherry water, sweetened with peony, clove and gillyflower syrup. For a week's time after the fit give two or three spoonsful of black cherry water for it. Last of all let 'em wear a single peony root necklace. Note: Always avoid giving syrup of violets, but syrup of roses and succory together are ever good. This may be given to children of any age or to men or women. Syrup of oil of amber may be given instead of Mithridate.

Cure Fits

Ingredients:

Camphor
4 pints of water

Porous bag

Method: Take a penyworth of Canfer put into a Tiffiny bag and put into it 2 quarts of water. For a child 2 spoonfulls 4 times a day and older person oftener and more in quantity.

A Cure for all sorts of Agues

Ingredients:

½oz of Venice turpentine
Camphor, powdered
Mastic, powdered

Sheep leather

Method: Take Venice Turpentine half an Ou: incorporate it with as much Camphir & Mastick beaten into fine powd'r as will make it into a fine plaster then take it & spread it on a piece of Sheeps leather cut round & lay it on the Stomach & navell pritty warm a day before the fitt comes. Probatum est.

To Cure a Dropsy

Ingredients:

½ peck of ground barley
¼ peck of red sage
⅛ peck of rue
8 gallons of small ale

Method: Take half a Peck of ground Barley, make it into a Loaf, put into it a quarter of a Peck of red sage and half as much rue. Put them in the middle of the Loaf and bake it, then get 8 gallons of small Ale ready and when Loaf is baked and break it small into the Drink. Let it work together and stand till it is clear then drink it for Ordinary Drink.

Cure Madness in Dogs, Cattle &c.

Ingredients:

A handful of rosemary
A handful of marigolds
A pint of milk
1oz of madder root
Enough wheat meal to make a paste

Method: Shred the flowers small and boyle 'em in the milk 'till half is consumed with the madder. Then make it into paste with wheat meal. Give it to the dog in a morning fasting him for two days before the full change of the moon.

Cure for Rickets

Ingredients:

2 pints of cream
Chamomile

Method: Take a quart of Cream and boyle it to an oyle then shred a deal of Camomile in the oyle and boyle it very well. Anoint the sides and stomach of the party grieved with some thereof warm stroakeing it downward. This has been tried on young and old and never failed. The disease is known by the head growing big and the flesh of the body wasting and hard knobs growing on the sides. It is much in Children, sometimes in old folks.

Dr Carmichael Smith's Celebrated Remedy for Preventing the Contagion of Infectious Diseases, in Hospitals, Prisons, etc.
(1807)

Ingredients:

A pipkin
Some sand, heated
½oz of vitriolic acid
½oz of powdered nitre

Method: For this celebrated remedy Dr Smith was liberally rewarded by the British Parliament. It has been found of great use in preventing the contagion of the yellow fever; and, indeed, all kinds of putrid infection. The method prescribed is as follows: Put some heated sand in a small pipkin, and place in it a tea-cup with half an ounce of strong vitriolic acid: when it becomes a little warm, add to it half an ounce of purified nitre in powder; stirring the mixture with a slip of glass, or the small end of a tobacco pipe. This process should be repeated, from time to time; the pipkin being set over a lamp, or one of the regular fumigating lamps for the purpose used. This has so often been tried with success, in infirmaries, gaols, &c. at land, and in hospital and other ships, that it is held to possess a specific power on putrid contagion, gaol fevers, &c.

Epileptic Electuary for the Cure of Falling Fits, Hysterics, and Even St. Vitus' Dance
(1807)

Ingredients:

6 drams of powdered Peruvian bark
2 drams of pulverized Virginian snakeroot
Syrup of peony

Method: Take six drams of powdered Peruvian bark, two drams of pulverized Virginian snake root, and a sufficient quantity of syrup of piony to make it up into a soft electuary. This is said, by a celebrated physician, to have been experimentally found a most prevalent and most certain remedy. One dram of this electuary, after due evacuations, being given to grown persons, and a less dose to those who are younger, every morning and evening for three or four months, and then repeated for three or four days before the change and full of the moon, absolutely eradicates epileptic and hysteric diseases; and also those odd epileptic saltations called. St. Vitus's dance, in which the unfortunate patient is afflicted with singular gesticulations and leapings, which have given rise to the name of that terrible disease.

Excellent Decoction for a Decline
(1807)

Ingredients:

2 gallons of spring water
½lb of figs
½lb of raisins
½lb of prunes
½lb of white sugar candy
½lb of pearl barley

1 stick of liqorice
A large quantity of horse radish and water cresses
5 lemons, sliced
1 pint of rum

Method: Boil together, in two gallons of spring water, till half reduced, half a pound each of figs, raisins of the sun, prunes, white sugar candy, pearl barley and a stick of liquorice, a large quantity of horse radish and water cresses, four lemons cut in slices, and a pint of rum. Take a small tea-cupful every morning and night; walking or riding' out, each morning, after taking it.

An Excellent Diet Drink for the Scurvy

Ingredients:

1 handful of:
  Cardoons
  Century
  Haymaids, otherwise ground-ivy
  Buckbean [otherwise menyanthes]
  Ground pine [on the endangered species list – illegal to pick in the wild]
  Sea wormwood
  The tops of St. John's worts
½ handful of:
  Broom flowers
  Rosemary
  Sage
6 gallons of ale wort

Porous bag

Method: Take Carduns, Centory, Heymaids, Buckbean, Groundpine, Sea Wormwood & Tops of St. Johns Wort of each one handfull, of Flowers of Broom, Rosemary & Sage, of each half a handful. Boyle 'em in 6 Gallons of Ale-wort instead of hops, then put the Ale into a Vessell & when it has done working put all the Boyl'd herbs into a bag, & hang it in the Liquor & in 2 or 3 days begin to use it for your Common Drink.

Excellent Pills for Jaundice

Ingredients:

1 dram of salt of steel
1 dram of wormwood
1 dram of steel
½ dram of soft soap
½oz of Castile soap
15 drops of oil of wormwood

Method: Mix the ingredients and make 70 pills to be taken 3 times a day for some time, 3 at a time.

An Excellent Receipt for a Violent Fever

Ingredients:

A handful of rue
2 anchovies
1 spoonful of bay salt
Some black soap, the size of a walnut
A whole head of garlic

Method: Take a handfull of Rue, 2 anchovies, a spoonfull of Bay-salt, as much Black soap as a wallnutt, and a head of Garlick – stamp these very well together in a stone mortar, then take one half & spread it on a Ragg and lay it cross the Ball of your Foot and lett it lye 4 of 6 houres. Then lay a fresh Plaister & it will certainly draw off the Distemper. This has cured Hundreds.

For a Lurking Fever by Dr Hulse

Ingredients:

8oz of Jesuit's Bark
1oz of snakeroot
6 quarts of white wine

Method: Put 8 ounces of the best Jesuits Bark & 1 oun: of snake root into 6 quarts of white wine. Infuse 'em 24 hours. Shake the Bottle 2 or 3 times in a day. Take a quarter of a pint of this morning & evening, poured off clear.

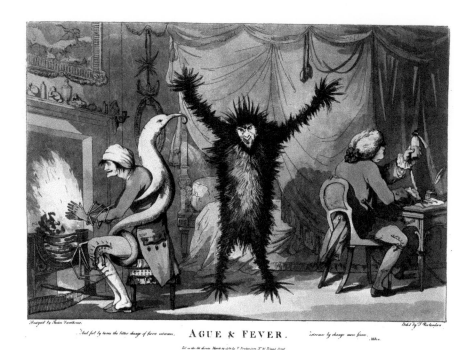

AGUE & FEVER.

29. Fever, represented as a frenzied beast, stands racked in the centre of a room, while a monster, representing ague, ensnares his victim by the fireside; a doctor writes prescriptions to the right. Etching by T. Rowlandson after J. Dunthorne, 1788.

Make Jelly of Grapes Very Good for One in a Fever

Ingredients:

A bunch of grapes

Method: Take the sowrest Grapes when they be almost at the full growth and fill one earthen pot with them. Cover them and put them over a gentle fire not to boyle but only to make the juce come from them, and as fast as the juce comes to the top poure it out and when you have a Reasonable quantity weigh it & put the equall weight of sugar to it & also put it on the fire only to be so hot as to meet the sugar thoroughly in it. Then take it off & shake it & let it stand to see how it jellys and then put it on again and warm it again and then keep it for your use: you may if you will strain it in a jelly bagg: this is good for the patient alone or with barley water if they like it.

Most Excellent Medicine to Guard Against the Plague

Ingredients:

3 pints of Muscadine wine
1 handful of sage
1 handful of rue
⅓oz of long pepper
⅓oz of ginger
⅓oz of nutmeg
2oz of treacle
1oz of mithridate
¼ pint of angelica water

Method: Take 3 pints of Muscadine Wine, boil it in a handfull of Sage and as much Rue 'till a pint is wasted, then strain it and sett it on the fire again. Then put therein of Long pepper, ginger and nutmegs of each the third pairt of an Ounce. Beat all together into a fine powder, let it boil a Little, then put therein two Ounces of Treacle, one Ounce of metridate and a Quarter of a pint of angelico Water. Dissolve the treacle and Metridate in the angelica water before you put them in. If you are infected take a spoonful or two of the mixture when 'tis warm. Do this both morning and evening in your bed and sweat after it. But if not infected, a spoonfull a day is sufficient, half in the morning and half in the evening to prevent infection. This is good also in the Small pox, measles, surfeits or fevers.

Mrs Browning's Cure for Gout

Ingredients:

½ gallon of new ale
1 pint of new mustard seeds

Method: Take a Pottle of new-Ale & put into it a pint of new-Mustard seed. Let it stand 2 or 3 dayes then drink a pint every morning, fasting. As you draw out one pint put in another. For the mustard will make it wast.

Mrs Cundall's Best Cure in the World for a Dropsy

Ingredients:

2 pints of white wine
¼lb of Castile soap
1 spoonful of olive oil

Method: Take a quart of white wine, a quarter of a pound of Castle Soap & one spoonfull of oyl olive. Mix 'em well together, drink half a pint at night going to bed 'till tis out.

Mrs Milborn's Cure for Scabies

Ingredients:

1 handful of:
    Sage
    Brown fennel
    Wormwood
    Rosemary
2 handfuls of rue
Strong ale (more than a pint and enough to cover the herbs)
1lb of unsalted butter
4oz of powdered brimstone (otherwise sulphur)

Earthen pan
Clean linen
Clean stockings
Clean gloves

Method: Take 1 handfull of Sage, 2 handfulls of Rue, 1 handfull of brown fennell, 1 handfull of wormwood, 1 handfull of Rosemary. Shred 'em small & boyle 'em in strong Ale 'till a pint is consumed, then strain it from the Herbs & put to it a pound of Butter well drained from the Butter-milk & not salted. Let it just boyle then take 4 oun: of powder of Brimston & mix it well with a little of the Liquor then stir it alltogether & let it stand in an earthen pan till the next day then take all the Butter from the top & clarifye it then pour off the Liquor clear from the Brimston. Let the Person infected take every morning 4 sponfulls of the Liquor fasting an hour before & after it & at the same time anoint the Body by the Fire with the Butter, both morning & Evening. Do this 3 or 4 dayes together. Put on clean Linnen, Stockings, Gloves, when you begin. Wear that shift a Fortnight.

Mrs Milborn's Ointment for the Small Pox

Ingredients:

The caul of a lamb
Spring water
Clean cloth
½ handful of marshmallow roots
½ handful of white lily roots
Sugar candy
Juice of 1 lemon
A small amount of spermaceti

Method: Take the caul of a lamb new kill'd. Lay it in spring water 9 dayes, shifting it into fresh water twice in a day. Then take it out & dry it in a clean cloth & peel off the skin, & beat it in a dry cloth with a Rolling-pin an hour. To a pound of this Fat take half a handful of Marsh-Mallow roots wash'd, scrap'd & slic'd, half a handfull of white lilly roots, half an ounce of which, sugar candy finely beaten, the juice of one Lemmon. Put all these together into a pot close ty'd down, boyle it 2 hours in a Kettle of Water then strain it out into an Earthen Vessell & put to it 6 penny worth of Spermaceti & stir it 'till it is all dissolv'd. Let it stand 'till tis cold, then cut it into small pieces & work it together as you do paste 'till it is soft & all the knots broken. It is to be used as soon as the Small Pox is quite off. Every night rub the face over with it & in the morning rub it off with a piece of dry Flannell & not wash'd.

Peony Powder for Fits
(1807)

Ingredients:

The root of a double peony

Method: Clean the root of the double peony, cut it in thin slices, and hang it up till thoroughly dry; then pound it very fine, and take as much as will cover a sixpence for three mornings.

A Pleasant Cooling Water to Drink in a Fever

Ingredients:

1oz of melon seeds
1oz of cucumber seeds
4oz of Jordan almonds, blanched
Water
Double refined sugar, to taste
Orangeflower water, or rose water, to taste

Method: Take Mellon seeds, Cucumber seeds, of each an Ounce, Jorden Almonds, blanch'd, 4 Ounces beat 'em together in a stone morter. When 'tis half beaton put in a little water several times 'till you have us'd a quart, then put it to 3 quarts of water more & stir it well together, then strain it thro' a Lawn sive. Then sweeten it to your tast w'th double refin'd sugar. You may put in a little oring flower water or rose water to give it a pleasant flavor. Bottle it up & drink a wine glass of it when you please.

A Preservative against the Plague

Ingredients:

3 pints of Muscadine
1 handful of Rue
1 handful of Red Sage
1 pennyworth of long pepper
½oz of ginger

¼oz of nutmeg
4 pennyworth of Mithridate
2 pennyworth of treacle
½ pint of angelica water, either strong or small

Method: Take three pints of muskadine and boyle there in one handfull of Rue and one handfull of red sage untill one pint is wasted. Then straine it out and set it over the fire againe, and put there in one pennyworth of long pepper, half an ounce of ginger and a quarter of an ounce of nutmegs, all these well beaten together, and let it boyle a little. Then straine it againe and put there in 4 penny worth of mithridate, two penny worth of treacle, half a pint of Angellico water, either strong or small, whichever you like best. Take of this every morning one spoonful. If the party be sicke take two spoonfulls morning and evening. It hath been proved to be the best remedy against the pestilence, for it was never known that man, woman or child dyed of the sicknesse, if they took this in time.

To Provoke Urine

Ingredients:

½oz of fennel roots
½oz of smallage roots
½oz of marshmallow roots
½oz of parsley roots
4 pints of spring water
1 spoonful of marshmallow syrup

Method: Boyle the herbs in the spring water 'till a pint is boyl'd away, then strain it & let it stand 'till it is cold, then pour off the clear into a bottle & take 3 or 4 spoonfull of it at a time, with a spoonfull of syrup of marshmallows stirr'd into it 2 or 3 times in a day. If it be too cold for you, you may put in a spoonfull of white wine to it. N.B. it must be only the outward rind of the Roots.

For the Rheumatism, Gout & Dropsy by Mrs North

Ingredients and Method: Take the juice of Elder Berries & boyle it to an Electuary. Take the quantity of a nutmeg the first three mornings every month in a year.

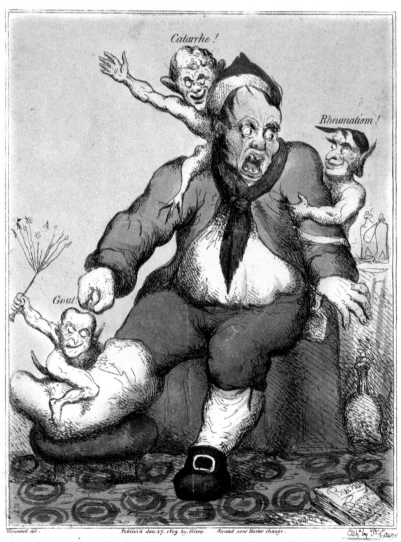

The Compliments *of the* Season *!!!*

30. A decrepit man screaming in pain from gout, rheumatism and catarrh; represented as three tormenting devils. Coloured etching by J. Cawse, 1809, after G.M. Woodward.

A Sage Pye for a Dropsy

Ingredients:

¼ of a peck of sea scurvygrass
¼ of a peck of common scurvygrass
¼ of a peck of Red Sage
4 Seville orange peals
Rye flour
5 gallons of ale

Method: Cut the herbs & peals together & bake 'em in a pye made of rye flour & when it comes out of the oven crumble it into 5 Gallons of working Ale & drink it for your constant drink 'till it is done. Let it be clear before you drink it.

For St. Anthony's fire

Ingredients:

1 handful of sage
1 handful of rue
1 handful of wormwood

Method: Boyle the sage, rue and wormwood in a quart of water to a pint then strain it out & dissolve in it a piece of alum about bigness of a French walnut then wash night & morning the afflicted part with a feather, letting it dry in by the Fire.

For Stoppage in the Water

Ingredients:

Inward rind of a great many pigeons' gizzards
Rhenish wine

Method: Take the inward rind of a great many Pigeons Gizzards and dry them in an oven, not wash them but scrape the Gravel from them and when they are dry beat them to powder and give as much as will lie upon a groat in Rhenish Wine 3 or 4 times a day. This has made persons make water and given them ease presently.

To Treat Worms

Ingredients:

½oz of senna
½lb of treacle
¼ pint of single tansy water

Method: Take half an ounce of Seana, beaten and sifted very fine, and half a Pound of Treakel and half a Gill of Single Tanse water, and Take 3 tea spoonfulls in a Morning.

For the Wind in the Veins or Elsewhere

Ingredients:

An equal quantity of
    Powder of liquorice
    Caraway seeds
    Sugar candy
A third of the above quantity of
Powdered rhubarb
    Pulverized cream of tartar

Method: Beat the liquorish powder, caraway seeds & sugar candy small and to your tast to which add rubarb beat to powder a third part or more with as much cream of tartar, pulverized: put this compound in a box, keep it in your pocket & take as much of it as will lye on a sixpence thrice in a day for a week together. It will gently purge you, cool the blood and expel the wind out of the veins and body. This has helpen those that have not been able to go. Take care you do not git cold in takeing it, but keep moderat warm.

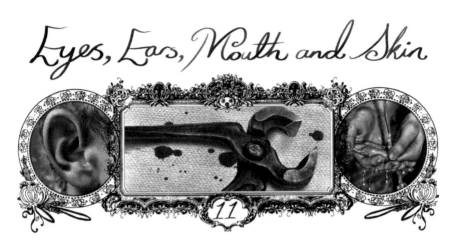

Aunt Dawg's Wash for the Teeth

Ingredients:

1½oz of mastic powder
2 drams of powder of olibanum
2 drams of powder of alum

Method: Mix 'em in a pint of white wine. Shake the Bottle when you use it.

Cure a Canker or Sore Mouth

Ingredients:

1 fresh egg
Honey
1½ drams of raw alum, powdered
1 dram of ginger, grated
1 dram of alum, burnt and powdered

Method: Take a new Lay'd Egg & break a hole in the top of it. Put out the white yolk & all then take the film or skin quite out & fill it halfe full w'th pure honey, a Drahm & halfe of raw allom beat to fine poweder, a drahm of Ginger grated Very small. Put all these into the Egg Shell & boyle it on a Soft fire. As soon as it boyles up & the allum is melted, take it off & put in a drahm of burnt allom fine powered. Stirr it togethar & take a Little upon your finger & dress your mouth therwith where you find any sore knots or pimples. Do this every day. A drahm is three score graines.

Dr Colebatch's Remedy for Deafness

Ingredients:

Asarabacca leaves, powdered

Method: Take 4 or 5 Graines of the powder of asarabacca leaves in Snuffe goeing to bed. It has cured a deafness of 14 years standing but the Patient must keep warm as in violent purges 4 or 5 graines to be snuff'd into each nostril every 4th or 5 nights & 3 graines to be blown into each Ear every night.

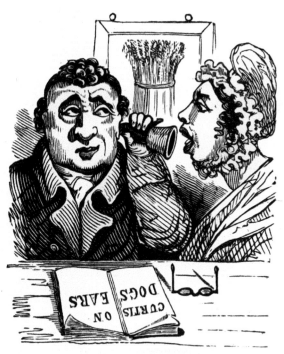

" I wish you a happy New Ear ! "

Elder Balsam

Ingredients:

Elderberries, enough to make 3 gallons of elderberry juice

Method: The berries put in a steam and so put in to an oven or a pan of water on the fire to drain of the Liquor then take 3 gallons of Elder berry Juce and boyle it to a quart in this manner: set a quart on the fire. When half a pint is boyled away, put into it a quarter of a pint more, and so do 'till the 3 gallons is all in and boyled to a quart but it must bee kept stiring all the time or it will burn.

For the eyes

Ingredients:

A like quantity of:
  Ground ivy
  Celandines
  Daisies
  A little sugar candy
  A little rose water
  A feather

Method: Take ground ivy, celandines & daisies of each a like quantity stampt & strain'd, a little sugar candy & rose water & put 'em together & drop it with a feather into your eye. It takes away all manner of inflammations, spots, webs, smarting or any other griefe whatsoever incident to your eyes. 'Tis approved to be the best medicine in the world.

Foxglove Juice, for Deafness
(1807)

Ingredients:

The flowers, leaves and stalks of freshly picked fox glove
Brandy

Method: Bruise, in a marble mortar, the flowers, leaves, and stalks, of fresh fox-glove; and, mixing the juice with double the quantity of brandy, keep it for use. The herb flowers in June, and the juice will thus keep good till the return of that season. The method of using it is, to drop every night, in the ear, a single drop; and then, moistening a bit of lint with a little of the juice, put that also into the ear, and take it out next morning, till the cure be compleated.

A Hand Wash

Ingredients:

1lb of bitter blanched almonds
½lb of raisins
2 or 3 spoonsful of ox gall
Sack, otherwise fortified wine
2 or 3 yolks

Method: Take a pound of bitter Almonds blanch'd, half a pound of Resons of the Sun ston'd. Pound 'em together into a past. Wet it with 2 or 3 Spoonfulls of Ox-gall, a little Sack, 2 or 3 yolkes of eggs. Mix these together.

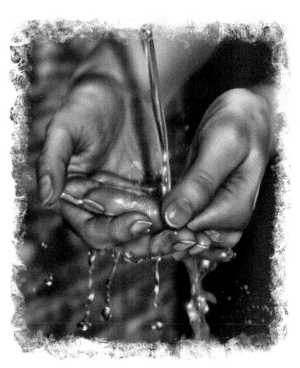

An Incomparable Cure of the Scurvy in the Mouth

Ingredients:

1 piece of scarlet cloth
A small amount of honey

Method: Take a piece of right scarlet cloth. Hold it to the Fire 'till it scorch yellow that it will rub to powd'r very fine. Then take as much burnt allom in fine powd'r & a little quantity of Honey. Sift the powd'r very fine & mix it with the Honey & rub your Gums with it morning, noon and night.

Lady Boothby's Excellent Water for the Eyes

Ingredients:

6 pennyworth of calminaris, otherwise calamine
2 pints of white wine
1 pint of white rose water
1 pint of rotten apple water, distilled
1 pint of eyebright water

Method: Tak 6 peneworthe of calominaris all in a stone. Heat it in the fire red hot. Queanshe it 9 timse in one quart of white wine and when you have done so beate the stone to powder and put it into the white wine. Then take a pint of white Roose Water & one pint of Rotton Appell water (the rotton appell must be destilled) and one pint of Eye bright water. Mix all thease together and when you wash your Eyes with it you must shack it & you may drop 3 or 4 drops into your Eyes. This is not only Good for any Rum but allso for a pearle in the Eye.

To Make Lip Salve

Ingredients:

¼lb of yellow bees wax
½lb of fresh butter
Rose or Orange flower water

Method: Take a quarter of a pound of yellow bees wax & half a pound of Fresh Butter & some rose or orange flower water. Shave the wax & put 'em together & set it on the Fire & keep it stirring 'till it is all melted, then take if off & let it stand 'till it is quite cold then take out the Cake & scrape it clean. You make keep it as it is, or beat it & put it in pots, whichever you please.

To Make Pomatum

Ingredients:

½oz of spermaceti
½oz of virgin wax
½ pint of oil of trotters, fresh drawn

Method: Take half an Ounce of Sperma Ceti, half an Ounce of Virgin wax, scrape the wax very fine, then take half a pint of Oyle of Trotters fresh drawn & put your Oyle & wax into a clean earthen white Bason & set it into a Saucepan of Scalding water over a very clear Fire & when the wax is melted put in your Sperma Ceti & which that is thro'ly melted. Then take it off the Fire & pour it into a pan of spring water & let it stand 'till 'tis cold. Then you must take it out of the water putting it into a clean earthen bason in which you must beat it for 2 hours or more 'till 'tis very white, then put it into a Gally pot & tye it down very close & keep it for your use in some cool dry place; you must not use anything of silver or pewter in making it. Beat it with a horn spoon, & when beating it you may put in a quarter of a pint of what sweet water you like best to give it a scent.

Mrs Hunter's Egg Salve for Boils

Ingredients:

1 yolk
Turpentine
Honey
Flour, to thicken the mixture

Method: Take the yoke of and Egg and as much of the best turpentine and beat them together as also an Equal quanttete of hunne and work them together then thicken it with flour so that it will spred.

Mrs Wroth's Cure for Growths on the Eyes

Ingredients:

Liquor that forms upon the surface of virgin honey

Method: Take a drop of the thin liquor that is upon the surface of virgin hunny, when 'tis candy'd, and drop it in-to the eye.

Opiate for the Teeth

Ingredients:

½oz of mastic
½oz of dragon's blood
½oz of bole armoniac
¼ oz of alum
3 or 4 spoonsful or clarified honey
Claret

Method: Take Mastick, Dragons Blood, Bole Armoniac of each half an ounce, Allom a quart'r of an ounce: let all these be beaten fine & mixt together with 3 or 4 spoonfulls of Clarify'd Honey. You must rub your teeth & gumms with it & then wash your mouth with Fair water or claret.

For a Pain in the Ear
(1815)

Ingredients:

2 drams of oil of sweet almonds
4 drops of oil of amber

Method: Oil of sweet almonds two drams, and oil of amber four drops; apply four drops of this mixture, when in pain, to the part affected.

Pommade Divine

Ingredients:

1½lb of beef marrow, well picked from the bones and filaments
1oz of storax resin
1 oz of benzoin resin
1 oz of sweet-scented cypress
1 oz of orris of Florence
½oz of cinnamon
2 drams of cloves
2 drams of nutmeg
1 white of an egg

Method: Take of Beef marrow a full Pound & half, well pick'd from all the Bones & Fillaments, then put it in a China or Earthen vessell full of spring water. Change twice a Day for 10 days, the tenth day drain it & let it then lay 24 hours in a Pint of Rose Water. Then put it in a thin Cloth to drain as much as it can then add, of storax, benzoin, cypress sweet scented, orris of Florence: of each one Ounce, of Cinnamon ½ an ounce, cloves & nutmeg of each 2 Drams, all these to be finely powder'd & extreamly well mix'd with the marrow, then put it in the Pewter vessell that is made for it & when it is shut as close as it can cover the top with a fine cloth & make a paste of flowers & white of egg to do round it, with another cloth over it that nothing may evaporate. Then put two sticks through the handles as small as will bear the weight of the vessell to suspend it in a Copper of boiling water which must not cease boiling one minute for 3 hours. Have boiling water ready to keep that in the Copper constantly at the same height. Take care that the pewter vessell touches nothing but the sticks that suspends it, then pour it through a thin cloth & let it run into the pots you design to keep them in, but don't cover it 'till they are quite cold which will be in two days.

Remedy for Deafness
(1807)

Ingredients:

1 tablespoon of bay salt
½ pint of spring water

Method: Put a table-spoonful of bay salt into near half a pint of cold spring water, and after it has steeped therein twenty-four hours, (now and then shaking the phial), cause a small tea-spoonful of the same to be poured into the ear most affected, every night when in bed, for seven or eight nights successively, observing to lay your head on the opposite side, by which the cure is generally completed.

Salve for Boils
(1807)

Ingredients:

A pipkin
½ pint of oil of roses
2oz thinly slice Castile Soap
¼lb red lead
2oz of ceruse [otherwise white lead]
2oz of hog's lard
4oz of oil of bays

Method: Put into a pipkin half a pint of oil of roses, with two ounces of thinly sliced Castille soap; and setting it on the fire, when the soap is melted, put in a quarter of a pound of red lead, and two ounces of ceruse in fine powder. Stir it well together, and let it gently simmer till it changes colour, and ceases frothing; then put in two ounces of hog's lard, and four ounces of oil of bays, stir it well together, let it simmer a little, take it off the fire, and roll it up for use. It will both break and heal boils, if spread on new linen, and applied twice a day.

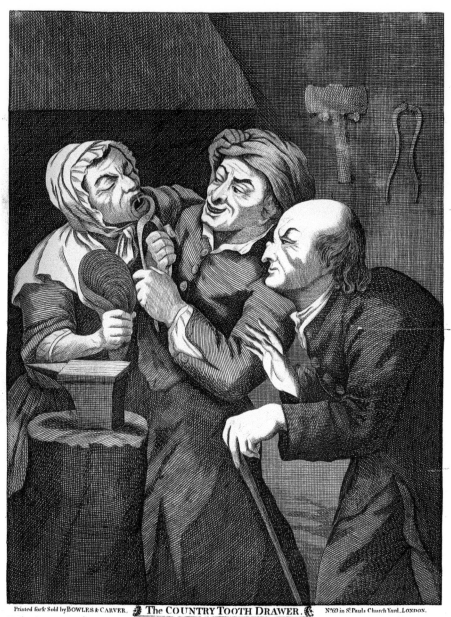

Printed for & Sold by BOWLES & CARVER. **The COUNTRY TOOTH DRAWER.** Nº69 in Sᵗ Pauls Church Yard, LONDON.

Why Dame how you hollow! and hold by my horn, | *That I hurt you, you neer shall make me believe, —* | *No doubt on't quoth Gaffer, and lets up his hand,*
I never heard such a noise since I was born,— | *Its easy, as drawing a pin from ones sleeve,—* | *Yet half of an hour is a great while to stand;—*
How you pinch up your hat and squeeze up your eyes, | *I challenge the Country for drawing you fool,—* | *And tho' you're surprised to hear my Dame bawl,*
You've broke both the drums of my ears with your cries, | *I've drawn tooth with prongs like a three legged stool,* | *Yet thrice round the shop is a pretty good hawl.*

31. A rustic blacksmith turned tooth-drawer extracting a tooth from an anxious woman patient. Engraving after J. Harris the elder.

Sir Thomas Haggerston's Cure for Toothache

Ingredients:

Tobacco ashes from a pipe
Brandy

Charcoal (optional)

Method: Take the Ashes out of a Tobacco pipe and mix them with Brandy 'till they are thick like a Paste then take some of it and Chomp it where the Toothachs but Swallow none down, still takeing fresh till the paine be gone. If you can get none out of a pipe take Tobacco and burn it upon Charcoal on a Clean Hearth 'till it comes to Ashes and so mix it as before.

For a Stinking Breath

Ingredients:

Coriander seeds
Sack, otherwise fortified wine

Method: Boyle Coriander seeds in Sack & drink it every morning fasting.

A Syrup to Kill a Canker in the Mouth

Ingredients:

Herbs (a handful of each):
    Grace
    Red Sage
    Honey Suckle Leaves
    Rosemary Tops
Burnt Alum, finely beaten
Honey
Any syrup, as preferred

Method: Stamp the herbs all together and then strain out all the juice and take a good quantity of burnt alum. Take also a quantity of honey and put 'em into your juice making it pretty thick. Stir it well and put into a pot and keep it closed. And when you use it rub the gums and sore places with it. You may wash your mouth first with water and then rub it with syrup (any of 'em will do it). The water will heal sore breasts that have a canker if you warm it and wash the breast with it when 'tis sore.

Water for the Eyes

Ingredients:

3 drams of tutty
3 drams of aloes
2 drams of white sugar
6oz of rose water
6oz of white wine

Method: Mix the ingredients and in a glass bottle close stopped, set it in the sun for a month, shaking it every day. At last being settled, decant & keep it for use.

This is such a wonderfull thing for there is few equall to it. It has caused those that have been totally blind for several years & alltho' very aged, made them see to read the smallest print by only washing with it morning, noon & night for a few weeks together.

Mental and Emotional Troubles

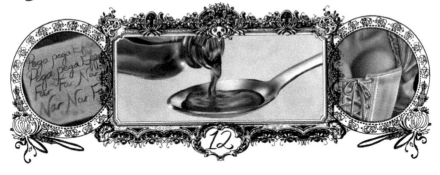

The Best Thing in the World for Languishing Spirits or Fatigue after a Journey

Ingredients:

½ pint of white wine
The yolk of a new laid egg
A little sugar
1 or 2 drops of cinnamon oil

Method: Take half a pint of white wine, put to it the yolk of a new laid egg or a little sugar, brew 'em together & put in one Drop or two of Oyl of Cynnamon, drink it off.

To Cure a Mad Dog

Ingredients:

1 handful of rue
1 handful of the bark of a box tree
Wormwood
Ale, plus extra for serving (optional)
Wheat flour

Milk, for serving (optional)
Butter

Hot brick, for baking on
Charm, prepared as below

Method: Take a handfull of Rue, a handfull of the Bark of a Box tree, and a small quantity of Wormewoode. Beete them & stampe them in Ale one houer or more, then mix the saide Ale with wheate flower. Make them into Cakes & bake them on a hote bricke & when you woulde youse them steepe the cakse all night in Ale. Next day geave it warme – geve in milke or else in Ale. One cake for one Creature.

NOTE: This Charme is to be writ' in paper and rold up in a peese of Buter and given to the Cre'r [creature] the Day before you give the Medic'n:

Pega pega Effema
Pega pega Effema
Far Far Nar Nar
Nar Nar far far

Dr George Cheyne's Cordial for Low Spirits, Fainting, Oppressions, Stomach Sickness, Headaches and Vapours

Ingredients:

6oz of chamomile flower water
1½oz of compound gentian water
1½oz of wormwood water
2 drams of:
    Compound spirit of lavender
    Sal volatile
    Tincture of castor
    Gum ammoniac, dissolved
1 dram of tincture of snakeweed
1 dram of tincture of the species diambra

10 drops of:
   Lavender oil
   Juniper oil
   Nutmeg oil
1 yolk

Method: Take of Simple Chamomile Flower water 6 Oun, Compound Gentian & Wormwood waters, each an Oun: & Half, Compound Spirit of Lavander, Sal Volatile, Tincture of Castor & Gum Ammoniack, dissolved in some simple water, each 2 Drams, Tincture of Snakweed & Tincture of the Species Diambra, each a Dram, The Chimicall Oyles of Lavender, Juniper & nutmeg, each 10 drops, mix'd with a bit of the yolk of an Egg to make the whole uniform. Two 3 or 4 Spoonfulls of this is present help in such Cases.

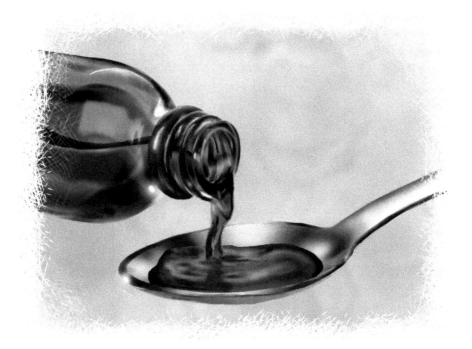

Dr Radcliffe's Famous Diet Drink for Sharp Humours
(1807)

Ingredients:

1½oz of China root
1½oz of eringo root
1½oz of sarsaparilla
½oz of ivory
½oz of hartshorn
1 dram of maidenhair
1 gallon of water

Method: Boil an ounce and a half each of China root, eringo root, and sarsaparilla; half an ounce each of ivory and hartshorn; and, a dram of maiden-hair; in a gallon of water, till it comes to two quarts. Drink it frequently, with a little milk or wine.

For Vapours or any Sudden Surprise

Ingredients:

2 spoonsful of water
1 spoonful of vinegar

Method: Give these to the surprised person immediately.

German Method of Preventing Hysterics
(1815)

Ingredients:

Caraway seeds, finely pounded
Small amount of ginger and salt
Bread and butter

Method: Caraway seeds, finely pounded, with a small proportion of ginger and salt, spread upon bread and butter, and eaten every day, especially early in the morning, and at night, before going to bed, are successfully used in Germany, as a domestic remedy against hysterics.

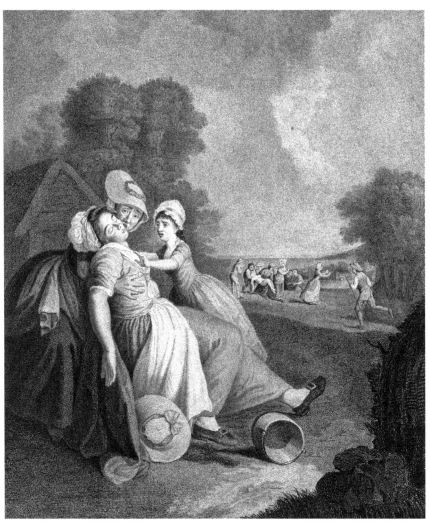

32. Engraving by W. Sedgwick after E. Penny.

To Make an Excellent Smelling Bottle
(1815)

Ingredients:

Sal ammoniac
Unslaked lime
Essence of bergamot
Ether, optional

Method: Take an equal quantity of sal-ammoniac and unslaked lime, pound them separate, then mix and put them in a bottle to smell to. Before you put in the above, drop two or three drops of the essence of burgamot into the bottle, then cork it close. A drop or two of ether, added to the same, will greatly improve it.

Mustard Whey, for a Palsy and Nervous Disorders
(1807)

Ingredients:

½ pint of boiling milk
1 tablespoons of mustard

Method: Turn half a pint of boiling milk, by putting in a table-spoonful of made mustard. Strain the whey from the curd, through a sieve, and drink it in bed. This will give a generous and glowing warmth, the whey thus conveying the mustard into the constitution, Dr, Stephen Hales says, that he knew a woman who had a great degree of numbness all over her remarkably relieved with two does only, and mentions several instances where it had done good in nervous cases, and in palsy, greatly abating the malady and prolonging life.

Powder for Vapours Occasioned by Wind
(1807)

Ingredients:

1oz of tormential
1oz of alexander roots
1oz of bay leaves
1oz of anise seeds
1oz of fennel seeds

Method: Beat to a fine powder one ounce each of tormentil and alexander roots, bay leaves, and anise and fennel seeds. Sift them through a fine sieve, mix them well together, and take half a spoonful just before eating. This is said to have cured a person who had many years tried other medicines.

Russian Remedy for a Vertigo
(1807)

Ingredients:

1oz of anodyne mineral liquor
1oz of liquid laudanum
1oz spirit of hartshorn

Method: The following is a genuine prescription of Roggers, Physician General to the Russian Navy. Mix half an ounce each of Hoffman's anodyne mineral liquor, Sydenham's liquid laudanum, and succinated spirit of hartshorn. The dose is fifteen drops, to be taken in the morning.

Wounds, Aches and Sores

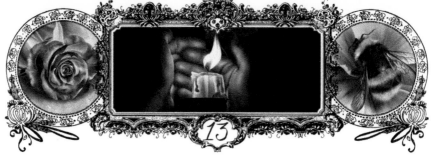

Admirable Ointment for Burns, Scalds, Cuts, Bruises, etc
(1807)

Ingredients:

1 well-glazed pipkin
4oz of olive oil
¼oz white lead
4oz bees wax
¼oz of camphor
Some white paper
Gallipots

Method: Set over the fire, in a well glazed pipkin, four ounces of the best olive oil; and, when it boils, put in a quarter of an ounce of the best white lead, very finely powdered and sifted, stirring it with a wooden spoon till it is of a light brown colour: then add four ounces of yellow bees wax cut in small pieces; and keep it stirring, till it is all melted and well mixed together. Take it off the fire, and continue stirring till it gets a little cool; then throw in a quarter of an ounce of camphor, cut or pounded in small bits, and cover it close over with white paper for a short time. Afterward, stirring it up, put it into gallipots; and let it be well secured with bladder, to keep out the air. This excellent ointment is to be spread on linen cloth, and applied to the part affected, the plaister should be changed every twelve or twenty-four hours, as occasion may require. Great care must be taken not to let the air get to the wound. It is said also to relieve pains in the ear.

Cephalic Snuff
(1807)

Ingredients:

½oz of sage
½oz of rosemary
½oz of lilies of the valley
½oz of the tops of sweet marjoram
1 dram:
    asarabacca root
    Lavender flowers
    Nutmeg

Method: Take half an ounce each of sage, rosemary, lilies of the valley, and the tops of sweet marjoram, with a dram each of asarabacca root, lavender flowers, and nutmeg. Reduce the whole to a fine powder; and take it like common snuff, as often as may be necessary for the relief of the head, &c. There are many more powerful cephalic snuffs, for particular medicinal purposes, but few so generally useful, agreeable, and innocent, to be used at pleasure.

To Cure a Bruise in the Eye
(1815)

Ingredients:

Conserve of red roses
1 rotten apple
Thin cambric

Method: Take conserve of red roses, and also a rotten apple, put them in a fold of thin cambric, apply it to the eye, and it will draw the bruise out.

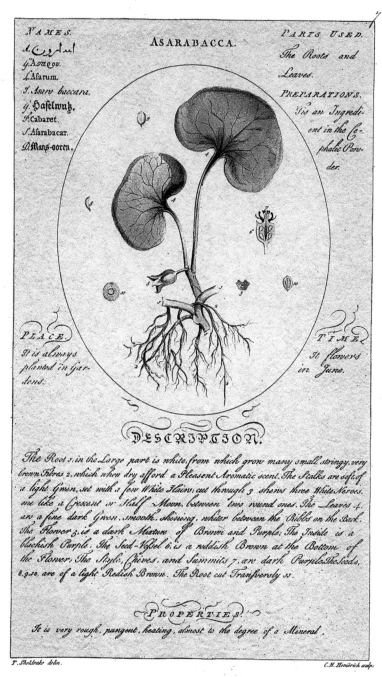

33. Asarabacca (Asarum europaeum L.): flowering stem with separate floral segments and cross-sections of the stem and a description of the plant and its uses. Line engraving by C.H. Hemerich, c.1759, after T. Sheldrake.

Cure for a Strain in the Back
(1807)

Ingredients:

4 tablespoons of white wine vinegar
Yolk of an egg
30 drops of oil or spirit of turpentine

Method: Beat up well four table-spoonfuls of white wine vinegar with the yolk of an egg; then add thirty drops of oil or spirit of turpentine. Mix them thoroughly, and drink the whole on going to bed at night. This dose, three times repeated, is stated to be an infallible cure.

The Cure for Sciatica, Dropsy and Rheumatism Evil

Ingredients:

¾oz of powdered pine apples
½oz of powdered acorns
½oz of powdered liquorice
¼oz of beaten ginger
¼oz of quicksilver, otherwise mercury
1 pint of warm ale
Honey
Gruel made with water

Charcoal fire
Dry, warm cloths

Method: Take 3 quart of an Ounce of powder of Pine Apples, half an ounce of powder of Acorns, half an Ounce of powd'r of Liquorish, a quart'r of an Ounce of Beaten-Ginger, quart'r of an Ounce of Quicksilver. Put all these into a clean charcoal fire & swallow the smoak of it as long as you can. After that lye down in a Bed wrap'd up in the same Blankets takeing a pint of warm ale & honey & sweat 3 hours, being rubbed with dry warm cloaths. This to be done for two dayes together then rest 2 or 3 days & do it a third time. The first day sweat 3 hours, 2 day sweat 2 hours & the third day an hour & half. After your sweating is over you may drink water gruell & Honey.

To Cure the Sting of a Wasp or Bee
(1815)

Ingredients:

Table salt
A little water

Method: It has been found, by experience, that a good remedy for the sting of wasps and bees, is to apply to the part affected common culinary salt, moistened with a little water. Even in a case where the patient had incautiously swallowed a wasp in a draught of beer, and been stung by it in the windpipe, the alarming symptoms that ensued were almost instantly relieved by swallowing repeated doses of water, saturated with salt.-The rubbing of the part stung, with a slice of onion, will give immediate ease.

A Diet Drink to Cure all Manner of Hurts and Wounds

Ingredients:

2oz of sarsaparilla
2oz of sassafras wood
1oz of china roots
1oz of tormentil roots
½lb of liquorice
¼lb of aniseeds
2oz of china
½oz of rhubarb

Two good handfuls of:
  Lady's mantle
  Marshmallow roots
  Sanicle
  Betony
  Columbine roots
  Agrimony
  Scabious
  Mouse ear

Colt's foot
Herb Robert

2 pints of white wine
2oz of senna
½oz of sliced rhubarb

Method: Take all the woods and herbs, shred the roots and the herbs. Put 'em into three gallons of running water, boyle 'em 'till half be consumed then strain 'em thro' a colander. Take the ingredients and put to 'em again two gallons of running water. Boyle the better half away, strain it hard thro' a coarse cloth & put the first and second liquor with the white wine and let it set. Scum it and when 'tis off the fire put it to the senna and rhubarb. Stir 'em together and cover it. Drink blood warm in quantities of half-a-pint thereof in a morning, at five in the afternoon and on going to bed.

How to Draw a Thorn or Splinter out of Any Part of the Body

Ingredients:

1 dry bean

Method: Take a dry Bean, chew it in your Mouth very well, then open the head of the place where the Thorn is & lay the Bean so chew'd on the place & in one night it will draw it out & cure it.

An Excellent Plaster for a Rupture

Ingredients:

1 gallon of the strongest wort you can make
1 handful of comfrey roots
1 handful of the roots of polypody of the oak, both well scraped
   and dried

Method: Boyle the roots in the wort 'till it come to a pint then strain it & rub as much of it thro' the strainer as you can, then let it stand 'till the next day. Then boyle it again 'till it come to half a pint, then spread it upon leather & use it as a plaster.

Famous American Receipt for the Rheumatism
(1807)

Ingredients:

2 cloves of garlic
1 dram of gum ammoniac

Method: Blend, by bruising together, two cloves of garlic and a dram of gum ammoniac; and, mixing up the mass with a little water, make it into two or three boluses, and swallow one every night and morning. Drink, while taking this remedy, a very strong sassafras tea, having the tea-pot constantly filled with chips. This is generally found to banish the rheumatism, and even contractions of the joints, after taking it a few days. It has long been famous in America, where, it has been affirmed, a hundred pounds were, a few years back, given for this receipt.

For a Headache

Ingredients:

½ a pennyworth of sweet fennel
½ a pennyworth of coriander seeds
½ a pennyworth of aniseed
½ a pennyworth of cardamom seeds
½ a handful of pennyroyal
½ a handful of century plant
½ a handful of elder-tops
½ a handful of mug wort
½ a handful of germander
1 pennyworth of chamomile flowers
2 quarts of running water
1 pint of white wine

Method: Take your sweet fennel, seeds, penny royall, centry, eldern tops, mugwort, germander and cammomile flowers. Boyle all these in 2 quarts of running water 'till it is half consumed, then strain your Liquor & add a pint of white wine to it. Drink half a pint Morning & Evening.

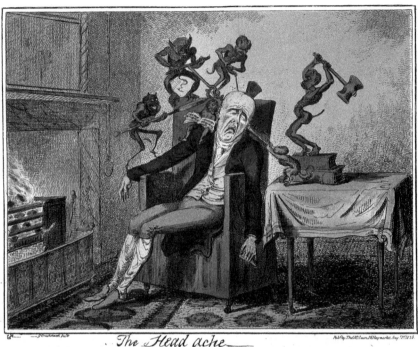

The Head ache

34. A man suffering from headache in the form of devils. Coloured etching by G. Cruikshank, 1835, after Captain F. Marryat.

To Heal any Cut

Ingredients:

Sixpenny worth of oil of spike
The same of train oil, otherwise whale oil

Method: Put them together in a glass. Drop it into the sore and bind it up.

Infallible Remedy for stopping Bleeding of the Nose
(1815)

Ingredients:

1oz sugar of lead
½oz of green vitriol
A glass mortar
½ pint of wine

Method: One ounce of sugar of lead, and half an ounce of green vitriol, to be triturated in a glass mortar; add to these half a pint of spirits of wine. Of this composition, young people, from ten to twelve years of age, are to take ten or twelve drops; patients under twenty years, fourteen or fifteen drops; and grown persons, twenty drops, four times each, in a spoonful of wine or brandy. Some very interesting trials, in the most obstinate cases, have been made with this mixture, with the greatest success. Remark.-No salt of lead should be taken internally without medical advice. It is a powerful drug; that is, if the proper precautions or proportions are neglected or exceeded, it is a strong poison. The green vitriol can have no other effect than to decompose part of the sugar or acetate of lead; that is, to convert the acetate, in part, into sulfate of lead, which is insoluble; and nearly all the green vitriol, or sulfate of iron, into acetate of iron.

M. Homassel's Account of his Cure for Burns or Scalds
(1815)

Ingredients:

½lb of alum powder
2 pints of water
Linen

Method: Take half a pound of alum in powder, dissolve it in a quart of water; bathe the burn or scald with a linen rag wet in this mixture; then bind the wet rag thereon with a slip of linen, and moisten the bandage with the alum water frequently, without removing it, in the course of two or three days. He relates, that one of his workmen, who fell into a copper of boiling liquor, where he remained three minutes before taken out, was immediately put into a tub containing a saturated solution or alum in water, where he was kept two hours; his sores were then dressed with cloths and bandages, wet in the above mixture, and kept constantly moistened for twenty-four hours, and that in a few days he was able to return to business.

To Make a Green Ointment called None Such

Ingredients:

½lb of bayleaf
½lb of wormwood
¼lb of rue
¼lb of red sage
2 handfuls of rosemary, dill, chamomile and lavender
3lb of mutton suet
1 bottle of olive oil
Parchment or leather and black wool

Method: Take bayleaf & wormwood, of each half a pd. Of rue & red-sage of each a quarter of a pd. Of rosemary, dill, cammomile & lavender of each 2 handfulls. Chop these herbs together, beat 'em in a mortar with 3 pd. of mutton suet from the sheep 'till tis all of one colour. Then put it to a bottle of best oyle olive. Let it be well mix't together, then put it into an earthen pot & let it stand 8 dayes close stop'd. Then boyle all together in a skillet upon a soft fire, being half boyl'd, put to it 4 ounces of oyle of spike. When 'tis fully boyl'd strain it into a Gally-pot, then tye it up close with parchment or leather & it will keep many years. It must be made in May. When you make it take heed you do not burn it. To avoid which 2 or 3 drops on a sawcer & when 'tis very green it is enough. Its virtues are as follows: rub some of it on your back, it helpeth the stone, chaff it into the Ears & stop 'em with Black wool. It helps all pains thereof, 'tis good against all Aches, coughs to anoint the stomach with it, swellings of wounds, tooth-ache, bruises, over-stretchings of sinews & cramp & stiches, sciatica, burnings, scaldings.

To Make Eau de Luce, and its Use
(1815)

Ingredients:

1oz of spirt of wine
4oz of sal ammoniac
1 scruple of oil of amber
10 grains of Castile soap

Method: Take of spirit of wine one ounce, spirit of sal ammoniacum four ounces, oil of amber one scruple, white Castile soap ten grains. Digest the soap and oil in the spirits of wine, add the ammoniacum, and shake them well together. The immediate application of Eau du Luce to many persons who have been stung by wasps, has caused the pain to subside in a few seconds, and after a few minutes all inflammation ceased.

To Make Balsamic and Anti-putrid Vinegar for Treating Wounds
(1815)

Ingredients:

White wine vinegar
1 handful of lavender leaves and flowers
1 handful of sage slaves and flowers
1 handful of hyssop
1 handful of thyme
1 handful of balm
1 handful of savory
1 handful of salt
2 heads of garlic

Method: Take the best white wine vinegar, a handful of lavender leaves and flowers, the same quantity of sage leaves and flowers, hyssop, thyme, balm, savory; a good handful of salt, and two heads of garlic; infuse these in the vinegar a fortnight or three weeks; the longer the better; and then it is found to be an excellent remedy for wounds.

To Make the Leaden Plaster Given by Lady Dering

Ingredients:

2lb 4oz of olive oil
1lb of red lead
1lb of white lead
12oz of Spanish soap
1 linen cloth

Method: Take 2 pound 4 oz of oyle olive, the best of good Red lead one pound, White Lead one pound, verry well beaten into dust, 12 oz of Spanish soape. Incorporate all these well togeather in an Earthen pott well glazed before you put them to Boyle and when they are well incorporated. When the soape cometh upward put it on a coule fire that is small. Continue sturring with a small Iron rod with a Ball at one end. One hour and half then make the Fire something bigar until the redness be turned into the colour of Gray which will be an hour and half Longer, But must not leave stirring till the matter be turned into the colour of oyle and som'what darker. Then drop it on a trencher and if it cleave, not to it or the finger, it is enough. Then take Linning cloath and spread it thin and lay on trenchers or boards when it begins to coole. Role it up for sear cloaths. It will last 20 years, the older, the better; you may make it up in Roles.

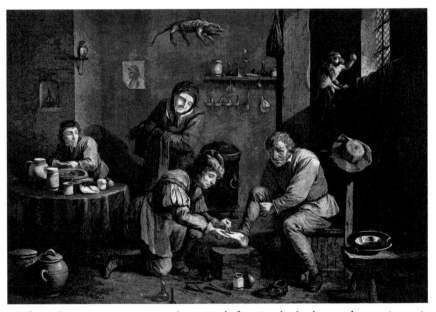

35. A rural surgeon treating a male patient's foot, in the background an assistant is mixing a concoction with a pestle and mortar in a surgery. Engraving by T. Major, 1747, after D. Teniers, the younger.

Oil of Brown Paper for Burns
(1807)

Ingredients:

A piece of thick coarse brown paper
Salad oil

Method: Take a piece of the thickest coarse brown' paper, and dip it in the best sallad oil; then set the paper on fire, and carefully preserve all the oil that drops for use. This is said to be an admirable remedy for all sorts of burns. Oil' of writing paper, collected in a similar manner, is often recommended for the tooth-ache.

For a Sore Breast

Ingredients:

4oz of lapis calaminaris, otherwise calamine
1 pint of white wine
2oz of tutty
1 pint of red rose water

Charcoal fire
Stone bottle
Clean linen rags

Method: Take 4 Ounces of Lapis Calaminaris in a piece, burn it red hot in a very clear Charcoale Fire & quench it in a pint of White Wine 9 times, it being every time red hot. Then take 2 Ounces of Lapis tutia make it 3 times red hot & quench it every time in a pint of Red rose Water. Then beat these Stones together into a very fine Powder & put the powder & water both in a Stone bottle shaking it every day for 9 days together once a day. Then take clean Linnen Raggs & apply it to the breast twice a day and every time you apply it it you must have fresh Raggs. Warm not your water you will take no Cold by it. In some Receipts it is a quart of White Wine & but a Pint of Red Rose Water or a pint & an half and the water shaked twice the day for a fortnight before it be used when the Powders are in it.

Speedy Cure for a Sprain
(1807)

Ingredients:

1 large spoonful of honey
1 large spoonful of salt
White of an egg

Method: Take a large spoonful of honey, the same quantity of salt, and the white of an egg: beat the whole up together, incessantly, for two hours; then let it stand an hour, and anoint the place sprained with the oil which will be produced, keeping the part well foiled with a good bandage. This is said generally to have enabled persons with sprained ankles, frequently more tediously cured than even a broken limb, and often leaving a perpetual weakness in the joint, to walk in twenty-four hours, entirely free from pain.

For a Violent Bleeding out of the Nose by Dr Fuller

Ingredients:

½ pint of vinegar
1oz of lead
1 linen cloth

Method: Take vinegar half a pint; sugar of Lead 1 ounce; dissolve. Fold a linnen cloth, dip it into this Liquor, apply it quite cold to the Region of the Heart, & as it grows warm, repeat it cold again. He says in a little while after, let the Flux of Blood be never so great it will most certainly stop it.

Wash and Fomentation for an Old Wound
(1807)

Ingredients:

2 handfuls of ground ivy
Roche alum about the size of 2 walnuts
6 pints of spring water

Method: Boil two handfuls of ground ivy with roche alum, about the quantity of two walnuts, in three quarts of spring water, till it comes to two. Wash the wound with it twice a day, for half an hour, bathing or fomenting with flannel as hot as can be borne by the patient. The use of this has been attended with very great success.

And Finally ... to Glue Anything

Ingredients:

A spoonful of brandy
A little isinglass

Method: Take Brandy in a Spoon & put to it a Little Iseing-Glass & boyle it 'till the Iseing-glass is dissolv'd, Then you may glew any thing with it.

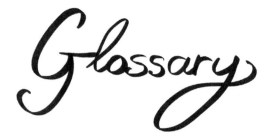

Glossary

agrimony	a herb long-used to treat wounds
alegar	vinegar produced by fermenting ale
alembic	a still used in distilling, comprising two vessels joined by a tube
alexander	a flowering plant, also known as horse parsley
angelica	wild celery
angelica water	the water obtained from boiling angelica root
anise	otherwise aniseed
asafoetida	a gum derived from giant fennel with a powerful smell
asarabacca	a flowering plant also known as European wild ginger or hazelwort
balm	an aromatic herb belonging to the mint family
betony	a grassland herb
bole armoniac	according to *The Country Gentleman's Companion*, published in 1755, this is a 'red, hard earthy substance, bought at the Apothecaries, and is of a cold and binding Nature'
borage	also known as starflower, the leaves are edible and are used in Italy to fill traditional ravioli
box tree bark	refers to a tree called common box, an evergreen native to Britain
brisket	meat cut from the lower chest or the breast of veal or beef
brimstone	sulphur
broom flower	a large shrub, often found on heaths, with bright yellow flowers

Canary wine	fortified wine from Spain or the Canary Islands
capon	a castrated cockerel
caraway	Carum carvii, a biennial plant also known as meridian fennel
cardo santo	a plant also known as carduus benedictus or blessed thistle, no longer considered edible, but traditionally used to treat colds
cardoon	a thistle from the sunflower family
Castile soap	an olive oil based soap from the Castile region of Spain
cawdle, caudle	a warm alcoholic drink, usually mixed with spices, sugar and bread
celandine	a flowering plant from the buttercup family, sometimes known as pilewort
century plant	an evergreen perennial that grows large leaves
ceruse	white lead, widely used in cosmetics in bygone days, but now known to cause lead poisioning and hair loss, amongst other health problems
China root	possibily the root of Chinese rhubarb
chocolate pot	a tall, slender vessel, similar to a teapot
citron	citrus medica, a large citrus fruit
cochineal	a red food colouring extracted from South American beetles
cockscomb	the crest of a domestic cock
coddle	to cook gently in nearly boiling water
codling	a type of elongated apple, used for cooking
coffin	an open-topped mould in the form a box for mixtures to be poured into
colt's foot	a plant from the daisy family
columbine	a short-lived shrub
comfit	a seed or nut or fruit that has been coated in sugar
cullis à la Reine	cullis is a strong broth for meat, so this would translate to broth to the queen. There is a recipe for White Cullis à la Reine in *The Lady's Companion* published in 1743. The receipt presented in the present book suggests white gravy as an alternative
diambra	a blend of ambergris, musk or other aromatics

dragon's blood	a dark red resin which can be extracted from various plants
elecampane	a plant in the sunflower family also known as elfdock or horse heal
eringo root	the root of sea holly
essence of bergamot	perfume from the bergamot fruit tree
eyebright water	a plant used to make medicine that appears in Greek mythology
flummery	a soft pudding
forcemeat	ground, lean meat mixed with fat, an ancient dish
galangal	an Asian plant of the ginger family
galantine	a boned dish of poached meat, served cold
gillyflower	the flower of a scented plant, such as the carnation
gizzard	an organ in the digestive tract of birds, among other animals
goat's rue	a herbaceous plant, often used in traditioinal medicinal practices
grace	a medicinal herb, otherwise known as herb-of-grace or common rue
green vitriol	another name for ferrous sulphate, which is a water-soluble solid that is used for a variety of purposes, included in medicine to treat anemia
greenwheat	also known as Freekeh, a wholegrain wheat roasted whilst still green
ground ivy	a member of the aromatic mint family, often mistaken for purple dead nettle. Also known as haymaids
guaiacum	a flowering plant
Guernsey sage	according to a book published in 1706 called *Silva, or a Discourse of Forest-trees*, this was held in great esteem
gum arabic	a natural gum from two types of Acacia trees
Gum tragacanth	natural gum obtained from dried sap
herb Robert	a common geranium
hiera picra	also know as hickery pickery, this is a medicine produced from aloes and canella bark

hogshead	a cask holding 52½ gallons, equal to 420 pints
hogs fat	lard
hoop	wooden hoop in which cakes were baked, similar to modern cake tins
hyssop	a flowering herb used to treat a cough
isinglass	a substance like gelatine obtained from fish for use in making jellies
Jamaica pepper	another name for allspice
Jesuit's bark	a source of quinine once used as a remedy for malaria
Jordan almonds	sugar-coated almonds from the ancient world
jumbles	biscuits dating to at least the Middle Ages
Kentish pippin	a medium-sized apple
Lady's Mantle	a flowering plant, believed to help with aches and pains
Laudanum	a tincture of opium
lawn bag	a porous, fine linen bag, suitable for cooking with, such as a muslin bag
long pepper	an Indian spice, also known as Indian long pepper
Lucatellus' balsam	a red ointment made of wax and turpentine
mace	a spice made from the outer covering of nutmeg seeds
madder root	a herb used in medcine, thought to be harmful to humans. Also used as a red dye in clothing
maidenhair	a fern
Malaga raisins	raisins made exclusively in the province of Malaga from the Muscat grape
manchet	good quality wheaten yeast bread, a recipe for which appeared in an Elizabethan recipe book called *The Good Huswifes Handmaide*
marjoram	a herb with citrus and sweet pine taste
mastic	resin from the mastic tree
meadowsweet	also known as mead wort, this is a perennial herb with a pleasant taste, common to Britain
mithridate	probably the herb Lepidium campestre and Thlaspi arvense

morels	wild mushrooms
mouse ear	a low-growing weed, commonly seen in gardens and hedgerows
muscadine	a grape native to south-eastern America
Naples biscuit	a type of biscuit, flavoured by rose water
neat's tongue	the tongue of a cow
nitre	sodium carbonate
oil of bays	oil obtained from the bay tree
olibanum	frankincense
Orris of Florence	the orris root produced by the white-flowered plant now known as iris florentina used in perfumes and soaps. Recorded in 1657 in a translation of *A Medicinal Dispensatory, containing the whole body of physick*
ox gall	bile, obtained from an ox
ox palate	the roof of a cow's mouth
pennyroyal	Mentha pulegium, a flowering plant from the mint family, also known as squaw mint or pudding grass
peony	a flowering plant
Peruvian bark	a source of quinine
pipkin	an earthen cooking pot
polypody	a hardy fern, in this case growing on oak trees
pullet	a young hen
quart	two imperial pints
race of ginger	according to Samuel Johnson's *Dictionary of the English Language*, this is a root or sprig of ginger
ragù	a sauce for meat created in the eighteenth century
red sage	native to China, this plant is noted for its highly prized roots, which are used in traditional Chinese medicine
rennet	curdled milk, traditionally from the stomachs of young calves or kids
Rhenish wine	a wine from the Rhine region of Germany, usually white wine
roche alum	a type of alum originally from Rocca in Syria

Roman wormwood	also known as Artemisia pontica, this herb is now used during the production of absinthe
rose water	liquid obtained by soaking rose petals in water
rue	therwise known as ruta, a shrub with a strong scent, anciently used as a herb in medicine
rundlet	a small barrel for wine of no defined size
sack	fortified wine, similar to sherry
sack posset	a spoonable alcoholic set custard
sal ammoniac	a white salt, ammonium chloride
sal prunella	potassium nitrate
sal volatile	an alcoholic solution used as smelling salts
saltpetre	potassium nitrate
sanicle	a herbal plant used in folk medicine
sarsaparilla	native to South America, a climbing vine grown in rainforests
sassafras wood	this wood has long been believed to possess special powers and has been used to cure all manner of ills
scabious	also known as pincushions, this is a plant from the honeysuckle family
scrag end	a cheap cut of lamb or mutton, from the upper part of the body, around the neck
sea wormwood	a species of wormwood, also known as old woman
sippets	small pieces of fried bread
smallage	wild celery
Smyrna raisins	Smyrna is in eastern Turkey and produced sultanas, which Sabine Winn called Smirna Currants
sorrel	a herb also known as spinach dock and narrow-leaved dock
southernwood	a flowering plant from the sunflower family
spermaceti	an waxy oil from the head of a sperm whale
spirit of hartshorn	a colourless aqueous solution of ammonia made from ground-up harts' antlers
spirit of nitre	a corrosive mineral acid, known as nitric acid
spirit of wine	purified alcohol, also known as aqua vitae
stone raisins, how to	by putting raisins in a dish and adding boiling water, covering them and returning 10 minutes

	later, raisins were softened allowing the seeds to be removed by rubbing each raisin between the thumb and forefinger
storax resin	a balsamic resin obtained from various trees of the Styrax genus and used in perfumed and medicines
suckery roots	a reference to this root appears in *Physick for the Poor*, a receipt book published in 1657, appearing in a remedy called *For the Dropsie and Yellow Jaundice*
sulphur, oil of	sulphuric acid
tacamahaca	a species of poplar
thin cream	single cream
tiffany sieve	a sieve made from tiffany, a thin muslin fabric
tormentil	a creeping plant, still famed for its medicinal properties
tutty	a substance obtained from the flues of zinc smelting furnances, consting of zinc oxide
twitch grass	a perennial weed
unslaked lime	white crystalline oxide
usquebaugh	whisky
venice turpentine	a sticky resin, extracted from the larch tree
virgin honey	honey that has not been adulterated
vitriolic acid	sulphuric acid
water germander	similar appearance to mint, the leaves have a garlic taste when crushed and is also known as garlic germander
Westphalia ham	ham from pigs of the Westphalian forests fed on a diet of acorns
wiggs	small, sweetened buns, often served at funerals in northern England. The name was derived from an Old Norse word meaning wedge
winter Savory	a semi-evergreen herb with dark-green leaves and pale flowers. It has been used in food and medicine
wormwood	a woody shrub used in medicine possessing a bitter taste
zedoary	a herb similar to turmeric